ESSENTIAL OILS FOR ALLERGIES

Be Smarter. Be Natural.
Be Allergy Free

By Mary Jones

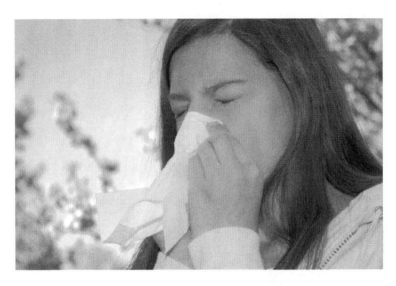

Over 60 Million people in the U.S. suffer from allergies and inflammation.
Did you know that essential oils are very effective when it comes to combating allergies
and relieving symptoms? They may also help boost your overall health without the side effects.

TABLE OF CONTENTS

INTRODUCTION

Do you – or someone you love – suffer from allergies and traditional medicine just doesn't seem to suit you?

Either it isn't effective enough against your condition or the side effects are having too deep an effect on your life? **Then maybe it's time to give essential oils a try!**

There are hundreds of thousands of uses for essential oils in healthcare, and allergies are an area that they are particularly effective. **This book will give you *all* of the information** you could possibly need in this area – what to buy, where to buy them from, what is suitable for what allergy, and everything else that you'll need to know – plus a selection of resources that will allow you to do some research of your own – after all, you aren't going to change your current health care plan without all of the necessary information! You won't find a more comprehensive guide to essential oils for allergies on the market. Read through all of the information included in the following chapters, and you might just find yourself willing to look after yourself in a much healthier way.

There is often a mix up with *'essential oils'* and *'aromatherapy'*. To clear that up right away, here is a definition of aromatherapy:

*"**Aromatherapy** is a complementary therapy that involves the use of **essential oils**. It may be used to help improve both your physical and emotional wellbeing."*

Below is a list of the **most common benefits** that people find from making the switch to essential oils. These include:

- *Very Powerful* – Essential Oils can have a healing effect mentally, physically, and emotionally.

- *Easy to Use* – they can be used wherever you are, and the methods necessary to take the oils are very simple – wear them during the day, diffuse them in your home, or simply keep them in your pocket.

- *Highly Effective* – they can penetrate the skin and affect the emotional center. So they can help you handle stress, anger or any other emotion.

- *Multipurpose* – you can make non-toxic green household products by blending essential oils.

- *Heterogenetic* – essential oils can have multiple properties, e.g. calming and grounding.

The more you use essential oils, the more you'll see that the benefits work for your mood and mind, as well as your body. So why not read on to learn more.

A QUICK GUIDE TO ESSENTIAL OILS

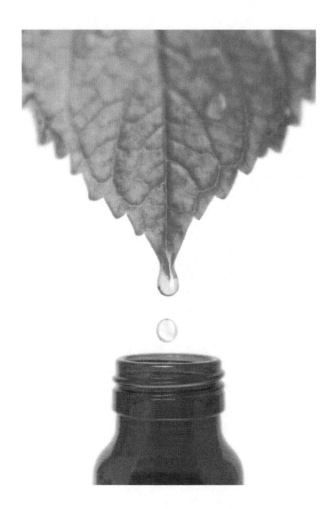

The National Association for Holistic Aromatherapy (*www.naha.org*) describes Essential oils as follows:

"The term "essential oil" is a contraction of the original "quintessential oil." This stems from the Aristotelian idea that matter is composed of four elements, namely, fire, air, earth, and water. The fifth element, or quintessence, was then considered to be spirit or life force. Distillation and evaporation were thought to be processes of removing the spirit from the plant and this is also reflected in our language since the term "spirits" is used to describe distilled alcoholic beverages such as brandy, whiskey, and eau de vie. The last of these again shows reference to the concept of removing the life force from the plant. Nowadays, of course, we know that, far from being spirit, essential oils are physical in nature and composed of complex mixtures of chemicals."

Put simply, it's a natural oil typically obtained by distillation and having the characteristic odor of the plant or other source from which it is extracted.

What you might not know about essential oils is *they aren't actually oils*! They don't contain any of the fatty acids that constitute what we would consider an oil.

Brief History

From all the records available, it seems that the Egyptians were the first people to use aromatic herbs and essential oils for religious as well as medicinal purposes. They are thought to have developed the distillation method which is still used to extract essential oils today. This system was passed down until it reached the Peruvian physician named *Avicenna* who is credited for perfecting it in approximately 1,000AD.

Since then, usage of them has dipped in and out of fashion. For example, in the Dark Ages, it was considered witchcraft, but these days, aromatherapy and alternative medications is *extremely* popular. That's because people are becoming increasingly inclined to heal themselves in a way that avoids all of the toxins and negative side effects of traditional medication.

2 WAYS ESSENTIAL OILS WORK

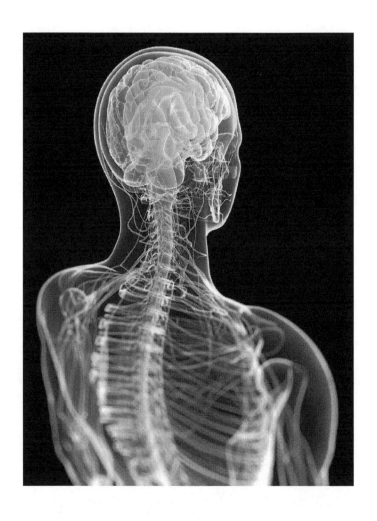

There are considered to be 2 ways in which essential oils work on your body. This is through body chemistry and the nervous system.

1. Body Chemistry

When essential oils are absorbed through the skin, they are working directly through our body chemistry affecting systems of the body. Each plant extract has chemical properties that are distinctive such as anti-inflammatory or cell rejuvenation. Tiny molecules of essential oils are easily absorbed by the membranes of the lungs and through skin pores and hair follicles. The chemical constituents/properties of the oils are carried in the bloodstream to all areas of the body. Essential oils bring on gentle physiological change.

2. Nervous System

Essential oils can have a healing effect both mentally and emotionally. The psychological benefits are usually obtained when essential oils are inhaled. Our sense of smell is governed by the olfactory organ at the top of our nose. Tiny cilia and receptor cells have direct access to the brain. The aroma sends an immediate signal to the limbic system of the brain. The limbic system is the center of memory and emotion. The oils can exert a powerful effect on mind, mood, and emotions.

TOP 5 REASONS TO USE THEM

Essential oils can enter the body in one of three ways:

- Applied to the skin

- Inhaled

- Ingested.

The oil is then absorbed and gets to work in the ways listed in the chapter above. They are great for a wide number of ailments, including anxiety, stomach upset, headaches and of course allergies – which is the primary focus of this book.

Many studies have been conducted by companies to discover the true benefits of these home remedies. The list of the **Top Benefits found** is:

1. They aren't toxic (if used correctly), so are extremely safe to use.

2. They are much easier to use than traditional medicine.

3. You can administer them anywhere, even at home.

4. They can travel with you everywhere you go.

5. They are very versatile and are proven to cure a lot of diseases!

Of course, there are also some **negative points when it comes to essential oils**, and these must be considered too when taking the choice to use them. The most prominent are:

- There isn't the same *regulation* as traditional medicine.

- *Limited research* – although there is more being conducted all the time.

- As with all medication, the *side effects* can vary so it's best to be aware of this.

When it comes to using essential oils, most of the negative effects or mistakes are down to simple errors and lack of knowledge, so it's best to ensure that you have all the information on hand before starting to use them. Aside for what is included in this book, there are many useful online resources when it comes to safety – so there is no reason not to be suitably informed.

PROVEN STEPS FOR BUYING ESSENTIAL OILS

After reading through all of the information in this guide, there will come a time when you wish to buy your own essential oils. While health professionals and experts will be able to help you, it is always best to be armed with your own knowledge to start with – to ensure that you're more likely to get *exactly* what you want.

When you start buying essential oils, there are a few things you will want to consider. **The most important three questions** that you'll need to ask yourself are:

1. What am I using the oil for?

2. What is the grade of oil needed?

3. What is the grade of oil wanted?

It is difficult to make a decision on this, without **understanding the oil 'grades'** and what they mean. As there is no one regulating body for these oils, this grade chart has been created to help buyers know exactly what it is they're getting. Note, that no government agency or generally accepted organization "grades" or "certifies" essential oils as "therapeutic grade", "medicinal grade", or "aromatherapy grade" in the US. There is no formally approved grading standard used consistently throughout the essential oil industry so the chart below is only provided for informational purposes.

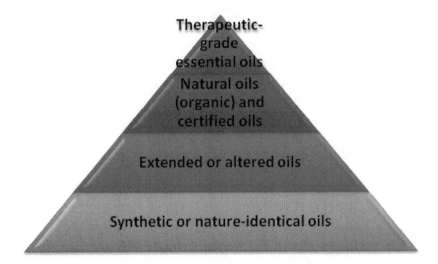

Therapeutic-grade essential oils	Pure, medicinal, steam-distilled essential oils containing all desired therapeutic compounds
Natural oils (organic) and certified oils	Pass oil-standard tests but may not contain any or just a few therapeutic compounds
Extended or altered oils	Fragrance grade
Synthetic or nature-identical oils	Created in a laboratory

For what we are looking at here, therapeutic grade oils are the most common ones you'll be considering. The **recommendation is to go with 100% therapeutic grade** wherever possible. Though these terms can be misleading, not all companies use these terms with intentional deception in mind.

There are many factors that make therapeutic grade essential oil, but all of them really fit into two main categories.

- *Environmental Factors* – Where the plant is grown; the soil type; fertilizer (organic vs. chemical); altitude, etc.

- *Physical Factors* – How and when the plant is harvested, how it is distilled and even how it is bottled.

These therapeutic grade oils meet stringent distillation and testing procedures and are produced with no solvents. They are costly to produce which means there aren't many high quality producers, but a little research will lead you to a reputable company. If you come across the company that uses the term *aromatherapy grade* or *therapeutic grade*, look for other key indicators of the essential oil quality and attempt to asses their particular intent in behind their use of the term. Some companies provide details on their site that define their particular use of the term. Whilst some companies do use these terms in a manner that is intentionally misleading consumers.

10 Tips You Should Know Before You Buy

Below is a great list of buying tips available for you that have come from real consumers. Read through the list, and keep them in mind when you're buying your own.

- Compare the smell of different brands of oils. Don't put your nose right up to the open tester and sniff - the undiluted oil is strong and can give you a headache. Instead, hold the lid at least 5 inches away from the nose and sniff.

- When comparing a variety of scents, take breaks. Sniffing too many different oils close together can overwhelm the senses and temporarily reduce your ability to discern differences in essential oils.

- Avoid buying essential oils from a company that prices all different oils at the same price. It may be a sign that the oils are synthetic or of lesser quality. The price of natural essential oils should vary greatly according to how much of the raw material is needed to produce the oil.

- Avoid essential oils that have been diluted with vegetable oils. To test, place a couple of drops of the essential oil on a piece of paper. If the oil leaves behind an oily stain, it has likely been diluted with vegetable oil.

- Choose companies that list the Latin name of the essential oil on the bottle as well as the common name, so there is no confusion. In addition, the company catalogue should indicate the country of origin and method of extraction for each oil.

- Choose pure essential oils over synthetic essential oils. Aromatherapists prefer pure oils, saying that synthetic oils may not have the same therapeutic properties as pure essential oils.

- Look for "pure essential oil" or "100% essential oil" on the label.

- Although the words "pure essential oil" are a good sign, it doesn't say anything about how the plant was grown or how well the essential oil was stored.

- Essential oils should be sold in dark amber or blue glass bottles. Clear glass can allow light to cause the oil to spoil.

- Don't buy essential oils in plastic bottles, as the essential oil can dissolve plastic and contaminate the essential oil.

Pure vs. Quality

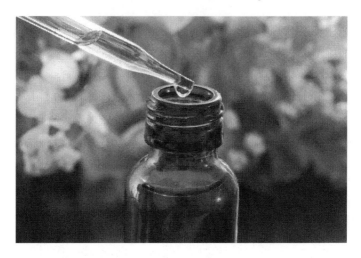

It is also important to know **the difference between 'pure' and 'quality'** essential oils when buying. Pure means undiluted, whereas quality refers to how well the product is made. There can be a bad quality oil, that's pure. For more information about pure and quality oils, check out the *NAHA* website at:
www.naha.org/assets/uploads/The Quality of Essential Oils Journal.pdf.

It may surprise you to learn exactly **how many plants are needed to produce essential oil.** In fact, on the extreme end, it takes 4000 pounds of Bulgarian roses to produce 1 pound of essential oil. Or a drop of peppermint essential oil is equal to 26 cups of peppermint tea. This just shows how much work and material is needed to make this, which is why a number of people believe that the higher the price of the product, the better the quality will be (but just to reiterate, quality is not to be confused with 'pure').

You could also do a little research into a company's standards and reputation, and make a judgment on the quality of the oil for yourself. The choice is yours to make but it's always recommended to discuss anything you use with a health professional or expert.

So now that you know the oil grade that you need, and the difference between 'pure' and 'quality', it's time to focus on the actual product required. Of course, that entirely depends on the allergy you – or your loved one – is suffering from, so we will go into detail on a variety of different scenarios – so you're bound to find something specific to you!

12 LITTLE KNOW FACTS ABOUT ESSENTIAL OILS

Here are some little known facts about the benefits of pure, therapeutic-grade essential oils:

1. Essential oils are the regenerating, oxygenating, and immune defense properties of plants.

2. Some essential oil constituents are so small in molecular size that they can quickly penetrate the tissues of the skin.

3. Essential oils are lipid soluble and are capable of penetrating cell walls, even if they have hardened because of an oxygen deficiency. In fact, essential oils can affect every cell of the body within 20 minutes and are then metabolized like other nutrients.

4. Essential oils contain oxygen molecules which help to transport nutrients to the starving human cells. Because a nutritional deficiency is an oxygen deficiency, disease begins when the cells lack the oxygen for proper nutrient assimilation. By providing the needed oxygen, essential oils also work to stimulate the immune system.

5. Essential oils are very powerful antioxidants. Antioxidants create an unfriendly environment for free radicals. They prevent all mutations, work as free radical scavengers, prevent fungus, and prevent oxidation in the cells.

6. Essential oils are anti-bacterial, anti-cancerous, anti-fungal, anti-infectious, anti-microbial, anti-tumoral, anti-parasitic, anti-viral, and antiseptic. Essential oils have been shown to destroy all tested bacteria and viruses while simultaneously restoring balance to the body.

7. Essential oils may detoxify the cells and blood in the body

8. Essential oils containing sesquiterpenes have the ability to pass the blood brain barrier, enabling them to be effective in the treatment of Alzheimer's disease, Lou Gehrig's disease, Parkinson's disease, and multiple sclerosis.

9. Essential oils are aromatic. When diffused, they provide air purification by:

   • Removing metallic particles and toxins from the air.

   • Increasing atmospheric oxygen

   • Increasing ozone and negative ions in the area, which inhibits bacterial growth

   • Destroying odors from mold, cigarettes, and animals

   • Filling the air with a fresh aromatic scent

10. Essential oils help promote emotional, physical, and spiritual healing.

11. Essential oils have a bio-electrical frequency that is several times greater than the frequency of herb, food, and even the human body. Clinical research has shown that essential oils can quickly raise the frequency of the human body, restoring it to its normal, healthy level.

12. There is a great test so you can discover if your essential oils are pure at home:

   Put a single drop of it on a piece of construction paper. If it evaporates quickly and leaves no noticeable ring, it is pure. If you have a ring left, then it is likely diluted by the manufacturer with an oil of some sort (this test will not work for myrrh, patchouli, and absolutes).

A QUICK REFERENCE GUIDE TO BOTANICAL NAMES

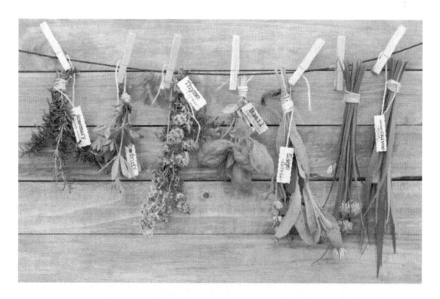

Many experts in the use of essential oils suggest that you have a much better chance of buying the best quality possible, if you have a good knowledge of the botanical names associated with ingredients. You can keep the chart below as a reference guide to ensure you're constantly in the know:

Oil	Botanical Name
Ambrette Seed	Hibiscus abelmoschus
Angelica	Angelica archangelica
Anise	Pimpinella anisum
Atlas Cedar	Cedrus atlantica
Balsam Copaiba	Copaifera officinalis
Balsam Peru	Myroxylon pereirae
Balsam Tolu	Myroxylon balsamum
Bay Laurel	Laurus nobilis
Basil	Ocimum basilicum var.Linalool
Benzoin	Styrax benzoin
Bergamot	Citrus bergamia
Bergamot Mint	Mentha citrate
Black Pepper	Piper nigrum
Blue Tansy	Tanacetum annuum
Camphor White	Cinnamomum camphora (Bark)
Cardamom	Elettaria cardamomum
Carrot	Daucua carota
Cassia	Cinnamomum cassia
Cedar Red	Thuja plicata

Cedar Leaf (Thuja)	Thuja occidentalis
Cedarwood (Atlas Cedar)	Cedrus atlantica
Chamomile Cape	Eriocephalus punctulatus
Chamomile German (Blue)	Matricaria recutita or Chamaemelum matricaria
Chamomile Morrocan (Blue Tansy)	Tanacetum annuum
Chamomile Roman	Anthemis nobilis or Chamaemelum nobile
Cinnamon Bark	Cinnamomum verum
Cinnamon Leaf	Cinnamomum zeylanicum
Cistus (Labdanum) (Rock Rose)	Cistus ladaniferus
Citronella	Cymbopogon nardus
Clary Sage	Salvia sclarea
Clove	Syzygium aromaticum
Cocoa	Theobroma cacao
Coriander	Coriandrum savitum
Cumin	Cuminum cyminum
Cypress	Cupressus sempervirens
Cypress Blue	Callitris intratropica
Davana	Artemisia pallens
Elemi	Canarium luzonicum

Eucalyptus	Eucalyptus globules
Eucalyptus Lemon	Eucalyptus citriodora
Eucalyptus Radiata	Eucalyptus radiate
Eucalyptus Staigeriana or Balm	Eucalyptus Staigeriana
Fennel	Foeniculum vulgare
Fir Balsam	Abies balsamea
Fir Silver	Abies alba
Fir Douglas	Pseudotsuga menziesii
Fir Grand	Abies grandis
Frankincense (Olibanum)	Boswellia carterii or serrata or frareana
Galbanum	Ferula gummosa
Geranium	Pelargonium graveolens
Ginger	Zingiber officinale
Grapefruit	Citrus paradisii
Helichrysum (Everlasting or Immortelle)	Helichrysum italicum
Hyssop	Hyssopus officinalis
Inula	Inula graveolens
Jasmine	Jasminum officinale
Juniper Berry	Juniperus communis
Khella	Amni visnaga

Kunzea	Kunzea ambigua
Lavender	Lavandula angustifolia or officinale
Lavendin	Lavandula x hybrid
Lemon	Citrus limonum
Lemon Myrtle	Backhousia citriodora
Lemon Tea Tree	Leptospermum petersonii
Lemon Verbena (Vervaine)	Aloysia citriodora
Lemongrass	Cymbopogon flexuosus
Lime	Citrus aurantifolia
Linden Blossom	Tilia cordata
Litsea (May Chang)	Litsea cubeba
Lotus White	Nymphaea lotus
Mandarin	Citrus reticulata or deliciosa
Manuka (New Zealand Tea Tree)	Leptospermum scoparium
Mastick	Lentiscus pistachius
May Chang	Litsea cubeba
Melissa (Lemon Balm)	Melissa officinalis
Marjoram	Origanum majorana
Mimosa	Acacia dealbata

Monarda (Bee Balm)	Monarda fistulosa
MQV (niaouli nerol type AKA Nerolina)	Melaleuca quinquenervia veridiflora
Myrrh	Commiphora myrrha
Myrtle	Myrtus communis
Myrtle Lemon	Backhousia citriodora
Neroli (Orange Blossom)	Citrus aurantium var Amara
Nerolina	Melaleuca quinquenervia veridiflora
Niaouli	Melaleuca quinquenervia
Nutmeg	Myristica fragrans
Orange	Citrus sinensis
Oregano	Origanum vulgare var.Carvacrol
Owyhee	Artemesia ludoviciana
Palmarosa	Cymbopogon martini
Patchouli	Pogostemon cablin
Pepper Black	Piper nigrum
Peppermint	Mentha piperita
Petitgrain Bigarade	Citrus aurantium var.Amara
Pine Sylvester (Scotch Pine)	Pinus sylvestris
Ravensara	Ravensara aromatic

Ravintsara	Cinnamomum camphora (Leaf)
Rock Rose (Cistus) (Labdanum)	Cistus ladaniferus
Rosalina (Lavender Tea Tree)	Melaleuca ericifolia
Rose Damask (Otto)	Rosa damascene
Rose Moroc	Rosa centifolia
Rosemary	Rosmarinus officinalis
Rosemary Verbenone	Rosmarinus officinalis var. Verbenon
Rosewood	Aniba rosaeodora
Sage	Salvia officinalis
Sandalwood Australian	Santalum spicatum
Sandalwood Indian	Santalum album
Spearmint	Mentha spicata
Spikenard	Nardostachys jatamansi
Spruce Black	Picea mariana
St Johnswort	Hypericum perforatum
Tamanu (Foraha)	Calophyllum inophyllum
Tangerine	Citrus reticulata or nobilis
Tansy Blue	Tanacetum annuum
Tarragon	Artemisia dracunculus

Tea Tree	Melaleuca alternifolia
Tea Tree Lavender (Rosalina)	Melaleuca ericifolia
Tea Tree Lemon	Leptospermum petersonii
Tea Tree New Zealand (Manuka)	Leptospermum scoparium
Thyme Linalool	Thymus vulgaris var.Linalool
Valerian	Valeriana officinalis
Vanilla	Vanilla planifolia
Vervaine (Lemon Verbena)	Aloysia citriodora
Vetiver	Vetiveria zizanoides
Violet Leaf	Viola odorata
Vitex	Vitex agnus castus
White Lotus	Nymphaea lotus
Wintergreen	Gaultheria procumbens
Yarrow	Achillea millefolium
Ylang Ylang	Cananga odorata var Genuana

BEST WAYS TO DILUTE ESSENTIAL OILS

Dilute, Dilute, Dilute!

LearningAboutEOs.com/dilute

Concentrated substances are rarely intended for use "as is" - and essential oils are no different. There is almost never a time when you would not want to dilute the potency of an essential oil.

Diluting essential oils is done by adding a drop (or more) of the essential oil into a carrier oil. This not only provides a good medium for the oil to absorb into the skin, but spreads the oil over a larger surface of your skin for more effect.

Another thing you need to be aware of with essential oil use, is dilution. Because essential oils are *so* concentrated, they need to be diluted so that they're safe to apply. The best way to achieve this is via a '**Carrier Oil**'.

These carrier oils are vegetable oils derived from the fatty portion of a plant, usually from the seeds, kernels or nuts. Example carrier oils include coconut, almond, apricot, olive, macadamia and sesame. Carrier oils should be stored away from heat and light to ensure their freshness.

There are considered to be five main *distillation methods:*

Water Distillation – This method is where the plant material is placed in boiling water. The steam and oils are captured and then separated out to produce the essential oil.

Water/Steam Distillation – This method is where steam and water are pushed around and though the plant material. And then the steam and oils are captured and then separated out to produce the essential oil.

Straight Steam Distillation – Distilling essential oils using the straight steam method involves pushing steam through the plant material and then picking up the essential oil.

Cold Pressed – This method involves pressing and grinding the fruit or seeds to extract the oil. Cold pressed oils retain all of their flavor, aroma, and nutritional value.

Solvent Extracted – Some plant aromatics are too delicate for steam distillation or too bound up in resin, so a solvent is used to make an extraction. The solvents used can be a range of substances (non-toxic and toxic) including hexane, alcohol, acetone, propane, etc. The solvent should be completely evaporated out of the finished product.

Dilution Ratios

The chart below indicates the **most effective ratios to use to dilute essential oils**:

Essential Oil Dilution Chart nourishingtreasures.com/EOdilutions						
Dilution	1%	2%	3%	5%	10%	25%
drops of EO for **1 tsp** (5ml; 1/6 oz.) carrier oil	1	2	3	5	10	25
drops of EO for **2 tsp** (10ml; 1/3 oz.) carrier oil	2	4	6	10	20	50
drops of EO for **3 tsp** (15ml; 1/2 oz.) carrier oil	3	6	9	15	30	75
drops of EO for **4 tsp** (20ml; 2/3 oz.) carrier oil	4	8	12	20	40	100
drops of EO for **5 tsp** (25ml; 5/6 oz.) carrier oil	5	10	15	25	50	125
drops of EO for **6 tsp** (30ml; 1 oz.) carrier oil	6	12	18	30	60	150

How much to dilute really depends on the issue you want to address. Here is a handy guide to take into consideration:

.25% DILUTION

AGES 6 MONTHS - 6 YEARS

Please only use for wee ones if you absolutely must. I personally prefer to avoid essential oils altogether for children under 2, and use hydrosols and/or herbs instead. If your child is sick, you may increase up to .50% if needed.

(.25% = 1 drop per 4 teaspoons of carrier oil)

LearningAboutEOs.com/dilute

1% DILUTION

AGES 6+, PREGNANT WOMEN, ELDERLY ADULTS, THOSE WITH SENSITIVE SKIN, COMPROMISED IMMUNE SYSTEMS, OR OTHER SERIOUS HEALTH ISSUES.

This is also the dilution you want when you are massaging over a large area of the body.
(1% = 1 drop per 1 teaspoon of carrier oil)

LearningAboutEOs.com/dilute

2% DILUTION

ADULTS

Ideal for most adults and in most situations.
This is also a good dilution for daily skin care.

(2% = 2 drops per 1 teaspoon of carrier oil;
10-12 drops per ounce)

LearningAboutEOs.com/dilute

3% DILUTION

ADULTS

Best used short-term for a temporary health issue, such as a muscle injury or respiratory congestion. Up to 10% dilution is fine, depending on the health concern, the age of the person, and the oils being used. (3% = 3 drops per 1 teaspoon of carrier oil; 15-18 drops per ounce)

LearningAboutEOs.com/dilute

25% DILUTION
ADULTS

Occasionally a dilution of this strength is warranted. This might be for a muscle cramp, bad bruising, or severe pain.
(25% = 25 drops per 1 teaspoon of carrier oil; 125-150 drops per ounce)

LearningAboutEOs.com/dilute

"NEAT" - NO DILUTION
ADULTS

Lavender is one of the few essential oils that can be used neat, on occasion, and only for short-term use. A bug bite, burn, or sting, might be a good reason to use Lavender neat. Just use caution when using undiluted, as some individuals can experience irritation or sensitivity.

LearningAboutEOs.com/dilute

It is important to bear in mind that it's always **safest to use the lowest dilution possible** that gives you effective results. Overdosing is an issue that is easily avoided by following this rule. As shown in the quote below, using too much essential oil can actually cause more issues than it solves:

Pure essential oils and absolutes are very concentrated. Many pounds of herbs, flowers, resins, or fruits are used to produce small amounts of oils...
Only small amounts of oils are needed to gain results...
Using too much essential oil can sometimes have a boomerang effect and aggravate, rather than soothe, symptoms.

colleen k. dodt, the essential oils book

5 ULTIMATE STEPS FOR BLENDING ESSENTIAL OILS

When you become confident in the use of essential oils, there may come a time when you want to create your own. There is an entire chapter in this book with recipes for essential oils to help with common allergies, so you can give this a go if you so choose.

Here is a great step-by-step guide to blending essential oils:

Step 1 – Finding Essential Oils with the Properties You Need

You can do this with a little bit of research. The Internet is a great way to do this, simply use search terms such as 'energizing essential oils' and you'll find many resourcing letting you know what you need.

Step 2 – Blending Essential Oils Based On Their Categories and Notes

Beginners often struggle with this part, but with a little bit of practice, you will quickly come to grips with what needs to be done. You will need to become familiar with the essential oil categories – a term which is used to help you get a great smell with your blended essential oils.

Essential oils categories are based on their aromas. Oils from the same categories tend to blend well together, but you can mix and match, as shown below:

- Floral
  (i.e. Lavender, Neroli, Jasmine)

- *Woodsy*
  (i.e. Pine, Cedar)

- *Earthy*
  (i.e. Oakmoss, Vetiver, Patchouli)

- *Herbaceous*
  (i.e. Marjoram, Rosemary, Basil)

- *Minty*
  (i.e. Peppermint, Spearmint)

- *Medicinal/Camphorous*
  (i.e. Eucalyptus, Cajuput, Tea Tree)

- *Spicy*
  (i.e. Nutmeg, Clove, Cinnamon)

- *Oriental*
  (i.e. Ginger, Patchouli)

- *Citrus*
  (i.e. Orange, Lemon, Lime)

There is also a suggestion of which of these **categories blend well together**:

- *Florals* blend well with spicy, citrusy and woodsy oils.

- *Woodsy* oils generally blend well with *all* the categories.

- *Spicy* and *oriental* oils blend well with florals, oriental and citrus oils. Be careful not to overpower the blend with the spicy or oriental oils.

- *Minty* oils blend well with citrus, woodsy, herbaceous and earthy oils.

Another term you will become very familiar with is **'*Notes*'**. The note of an essential oil is based on how quickly it evaporates. When you put a blend of oils on your skin, it will smell one way, but 3 hours later it may smell another way because some of the oils in your blend have evaporated. These notes are based on the musical scale and are referred to as top notes, middle notes, and base notes.

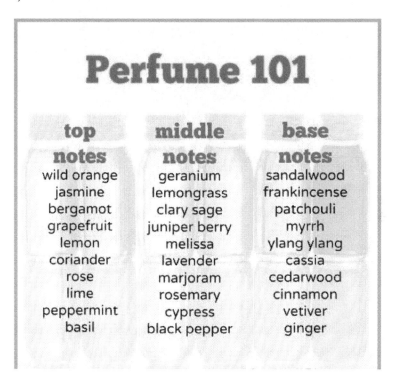

Perfume 101

top notes	middle notes	base notes
wild orange	geranium	sandalwood
jasmine	lemongrass	frankincense
bergamot	clary sage	patchouli
grapefruit	juniper berry	myrrh
lemon	melissa	ylang ylang
coriander	lavender	cassia
rose	marjoram	cedarwood
lime	rosemary	cinnamon
peppermint	cypress	vetiver
basil	black pepper	ginger

Most times, for beginners, it's recommended that you only *start with three oils*. A top note oil, a middle note oil, and a base note oil. The more comfortable and experienced you get with blending essential oils; the more oils you can add to your blends.

Step 3 – Blending and Testing Essential Oil Blends

Once you've narrowed down your oil choices based on what they're used for (step 1) and then narrowed them down again based on their categories and notes (step 2), you're ready to actually **start blending**.

It's recommended that you only **start with 10 drops** of oil total so you can test your essential oil blend without wasting too much of your precious oils, in case you don't care for it later.

Remember, you're only working with your essential oils right now…you are not diluting them with carrier oils yet.

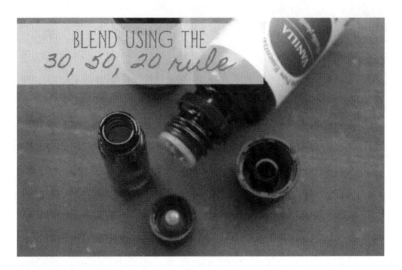

Another thing you may be wondering is how much do you use of each oil. The most commonly used rule to go by when creating an essential oil blend is the *30, 50, 20 rule:*

- 30% of your *top note oil.*

- 50% of your *middle note oil.*

- 20% of your *base note oil.*

This is because when you use your blend, you're going to smell all the oils together first. After a while the top note will have evaporated which will leave you with the middle and base note. As more time goes by your middle note will evaporate leaving you with the base note alone. Smell is very important when using essential oils with dogs, so this is very important.

Step 4 – Letting Your Essential Oil Blend "Rest"

This next step is the easy part. Once you've mixed your oils you need to set your new blend aside and let it rest for 24 - 48 hours. This resting period allows the chemicals and constituents of the different essential oils to mix and meld together, helping them blend better.

Step 5 – Testing Your Blend

This is the last step on blending essential oils. At this point, your oils have just finished their resting period. Now it's time to smell them and see what you think.

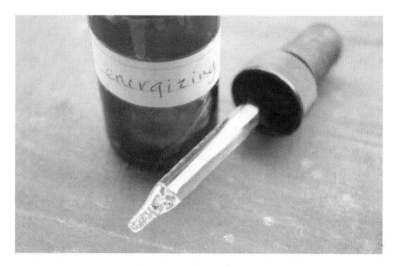

Next try **diluting some of your blend** in a carrier oil. Once you have got the blend right, you can make up more of the oil, allow it to rest the bottle it up to use as necessary.

8 TESTED BLENDING TIPS

1. When creating a new blend, start out small with a total number of drops – between 5 and 25. This will ensure that you waste less oil in experiments.

2. Start creating your blend by using only essential oils. Wait until you include carrier oils so as not to waste them.

3. Keep a notebook of everything you do, because when the creative juices are flowing you might forget exactly what was written.

4. Perfume sample bottles are great for storage. They're inexpensive and easily found to purchase.

5. Be sure to label your blends clearly. If you don't have to write everything out, but you need some way to decipher what you've created.

6. It is important to use the 30 – 50 – 20 rule when first starting out blending.

7. Some oils are stronger than others. Unless you want certain oils to dominate your blend, it is best to do some research on what you're using. The Internet is filled with online forums and resources which you can use to communicate with others.

8. After creating your blend, it is best to let it sit for a few days before making a decision about whether you love or hate it. The constitutes need time to adjust to one another.

GUIDE FOR STORING
ESSENTIAL OILS

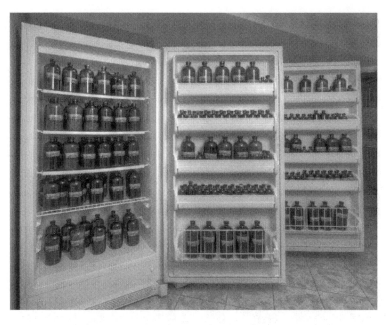

The way you look after your essential oils *will* affect their shelf life, so it's important to follow the correct procedure to save yourself time, money and effort. Here is a great *'Do's and Don'ts'* guide:

1. *Don't* expose your essential oils to extreme or rapid changes in temperature.

2. *Do* keep your essential oils packaged in dark, colored glass because this filters out the suns UV rays.

3. *Do* keep your essential oils stored in a cool, dark place.

4. *Do* use the refrigerator to store your essential oils if you have the space.

5. *Don't* let your carrier oils get too warm as this will compromise the quality of the essential oils.

6. *Do* consider using an aromatherapy box if you don't have the room in your refrigerator. These are specifically designed to keep your essential oils at the desired temperature.

7. *Do* replace the cap of your essential oil bottles immediately after you have finished using them. They are prone to evaporating and you don't want to risk losing them in this way.

8. *Don't* ever leave your essential oils near naked flame as they are highly flammable materials.

9. *Don't* ever decant your essential oils into plastic bottles as they will likely melt through it.

THE MOST COMMON
APPLICATION TECHNIQUES

So now that we've looked at buying, diluting and storing essential oils, it's time to talk about **proper application**. Getting this right is very important as it can help or hinder your recovery. There are considered to be four main application techniques; *aromatically, topically, internally or externally*, all of which we are going to examine in detail through this chapter.

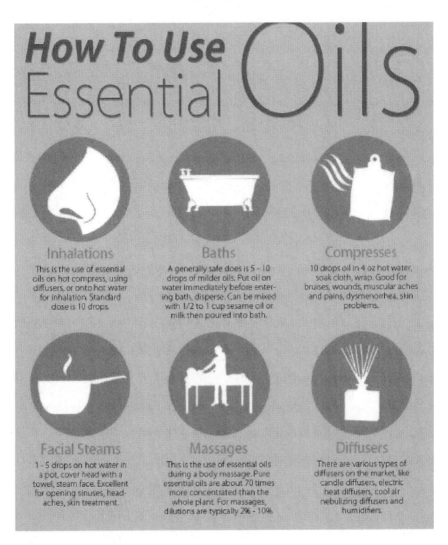

How To Use Essential Oils

Inhalations
This is the use of essential oils on hot compress, using diffusers, or onto hot water for inhalation. Standard dose is 10 drops.

Baths
A generally safe does is 5 - 10 drops of milder oils. Put oil on water immediately before entering bath, disperse. Can be mixed with 1/2 to 1 cup sesame oil or milk then poured into bath.

Compresses
10 drops oil in 4 oz hot water, soak cloth, wrap. Good for bruises, wounds, muscular aches and pains, dysmenorrhea, skin problems.

Facial Steams
1 - 5 drops on hot water in a pot, cover head with a towel, steam face. Excellent for opening sinuses, headaches, skin treatment.

Massages
This is the use of essential oils during a body massage. Pure essential oils are about 70 times more concentrated than the whole plant. For massages, dilutions are typically 2% - 10%.

Diffusers
There are various types of diffusers on the market, like candle diffusers, electric heat diffusers, cool air nebulizing diffusers and humidifiers.

Below is a guide to using essential oils correctly.

Aromatic

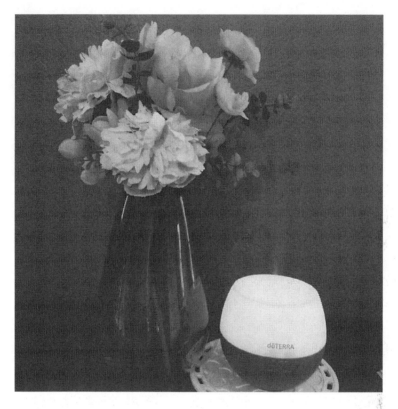

The aromatic application is the most widely used. This is because the positive properties of essential oils can be absorbed into the blood stream *through inhalation*. This method of application can:

- Be nurturing to the respiratory system, including the sinuses.

- Have a supportive effect on moods, the hormonal system, tension, etc.

- Increase indoor air quality or help protect against airborne contaminants.

- The positive compounds and their properties, once within our blood stream, can encourage our immune system response or promote wellbeing in a multitude of ways.

The methods for this type of application are:

- *Diffusing:* A good diffuser should use cool or room temperature air or ultrasonic vibrations to diffuse the oil into the air, which help the oil molecules remain air-bound for several more hours and do not affect the structure of the oil through heat, which can diminish the quality of the oil.

- *Direct Inhalation:* Directly inhaling the oil can be done by holding the bottle of essential oil a few inches from the nose and breathing in the aroma, or by adding a drop to the hands and cupping them over the mouth and nose. (For example, using this technique can be used with grounding or calming oils.) It is important to note that constantly opening and closing your bottle does exposure it to air and increase the oxidation rate, so diffusing is not only better for your bottle of oil, but you would likely use less throughout the day too. Some oils, such as Oregano or Cinnamon, should also be diluted before direct inhalation.

- *Indirect Inhalation:* Adding a drop to a handkerchief, cotton ball, small square of fabric, shirt collar, hair, pillow case, etc. can all be beneficial. (Try this with Vetiver when you want to promote deeper sleep!)

- *Hot Water Vapor/Steam Tent:* Heat a pot of water (not boiling), add 1-3 drops of essential oil, place a towel over your head while leaning over the water, and inhale the steam. (For example, try this with Eucalyptus for respiratory health.)

- *Humidifier:* Just like a diffuser, cool air humidifiers are best. Be aware that essential oils can damage plastic components over time, so choosing one made for essential oils is best. (Try a purifying oil to clean the air.)

- *Fan, Vent, Etc.:* Just like with the indirect inhalation, you can add the oil to cloth and place it in a vent or even in front of a fan. (A good use for this is Peppermint or Ginger in the car to calm motion sickness.)

- *Perfume or Cologne:* Smells good and is safer and healthier for your body (unlike normal chemical-based perfumes or antiperspirants). For perfume or cologne, add a 1 drop or a small dab to the wrists, behind the ears, or add 10 drops to 1-3 tsp of distilled water or alcohol to mist on the body or clothing.

- ***Natural Room Deodorizer:*** Instead of harsh chemicals to cover up odors you can add essential oils to your odor removing efforts. For instance, you can create a room deodorizer by mixing a half cup of alcohol (such as vodka) with a half cup of distilled water, and 20-40 drops of your favorite essential oils in a decorative jar. Then add 10 or so bamboo skewers (like the ones you use for kebobs) to the mixture so that they are sticking out of the bottle. They will soak up the aroma and spread it throughout a bathroom easily. You can also create a spray.

Even though learning how to use essential oils aromatically is probably the easiest and safest, it's still important to know your body, and pay attention to how it responds to the oils. Aromatic is still a potent use of essential oils. Too much can overwhelm your system, give you a headache, or even cause a reaction if you're sensitive or allergic to the oil.

Topically

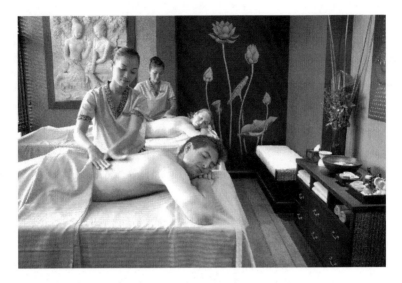

Learning how to use essential oils topically is a little more delicate, but still fairly simple. Please remember that although most essential oils can be used topically, *how* they are used will vary from oil to oil. Some come with precautions for dilution or frequency, but even those that don't, can still affect some skin types, causing itchiness or a rash if not used with care.

It is very important to **know your skin type**. Do you tend to have sensitive skin? Then always dilute, no matter the oil. If you aren't sure, do a patch test an area of your inner arm first. Start with one diluted drop, then increase an undiluted drop if the oil is generally safe for undiluted use in most people. And always use *one oil at a time*, so that if you have a negative reaction, you know what you reacted to.

Diluting never hurts! It doesn't decrease the effectiveness of the oil, and may help to increase absorption by preventing evaporation, as well as decreasing the likelihood of the skin reaction, so unless you have reasons not to, it's good idea to do so.

- *Neat – Oils generally safe to use undiluted:* This means you can generally apply the oil in question directly to the skin without any dilution. *However*, it's still a good idea to patch test your own skin first, just in case, or follow sensitivity guidelines above if you know you have sensitive skin. Also, because dilution can't hurt and can help, it's a good idea to do it anyway.

- *Sensitive - _Oils to be used with moderate dilution:_* This means that although some can apply the oil without any dilution, directly to the skin, those with sensitive skin, as well as children and the elderly, should do a patch test or dilute before use. Use a guideline of 1 drop per 1-4 oz. of carrier oil, such as coconut oil, or at minimum a 1:3 ratio (1 drop of essential oil to every 3 drops of carrier).

- *Dilute – _Oils generally safe to use with heavier dilution:_* **These oils are very potent**. It's important that you dilute these *at least* 1:3 and more depending on age and skin sensitivity, as they can cause irritation to any skin type when applied directly. If you're pregnant or nursing, use more caution or talk to your naturopathic doctor. I would personally avoid for children, although a high dilution rate may be okay in small amounts for a limited period of time. For more information check Dilution chapter.

There are some other **topical precautions that you should consider**:

- *Citrus oils* can cause sensitivity to the sun. It's usually recommended to avoid sunlight within 12 hours of applying topically, but Bergamot in particular can cause issues for up to 3 days. We usually will apply these in the evening, or to an area of the body that won't be exposed to the sun, or we avoid topical use altogether.

- Everyone is different and even the gentlest oils can still cause a reaction. If you know you're prone to sensitive skin or skin reactions, always test the oils highly diluted first, then with a lighter dilution, before trying undiluted if it's an oil that is generally recognize as one you can use "neat". Like I said above, dilution never hurts, so if in doubt, dilute.

- Even if you've used an oil before without problems or don't consider yourself to have sensitive skin, you can still develop a reaction to it with excessive use over the same area of the body. Try to mix it up when possible (alternating application locations *and* the oils you're using) and dilute as necessary. Because you may not know you have a sensitivity, this is why many say you should *always* dilute. You may feel comfortable not diluting some "neat" oils, but when in doubt, dilute.

- It's usually better to "layer" oils than to blend them. What this means is that if you're using 2 or more oils topically, apply one, then wait between 5-30 minutes and apply the other over it (instead of mixing a drop of each in your hand and then rubbing this into the skin). Mixing the oils is as much an art as it is a science, which is why we tend to stick to the blends a company has already created, since we know they are safe and effective.

The popular methods of topical essential oil applications are as follows:

- *In a Massage:* Massage is one of the most enjoyable ways to use essential oils topically. Massaging the oils into joints, muscles, and tissues is relaxing and beneficial. Always move toward the heart when working on the arms and legs and avoid a heavy hand, or moving over the spine or other sensitive areas, with too much pressure.

- *Over the Area of Concern:* The next option is to apply the oils to the chest, the abdomen, back of the neck, or directly over the area of concern (diluted as indicated). You can also apply to the energy centers of the body.

- *Over the Reflex Points:* But probably the best, most effective, and yet gentlest option for how to use essential oils, especially for sensitive skin, children, or elderly, is to apply the oils to the reflex points of the feet, hands, and even ears (still dilute as needed). The feet especially are beneficial because of how quickly it absorbs into the blood stream, but they are tough enough to make the likelihood of irritation much less if your skin is prone to reactions, and easy to cover if you don't like the aroma or if you're applying to a child and don't want them touching it (cover their feet with socks). The reflex points of the hands and feet also correspond to the different areas of the body by way of the nervous system. Learning how to use essential oils is made easier with visual guides to reflexology to understand which reflex points to massage the oil into based on the area of the body you wish to support.

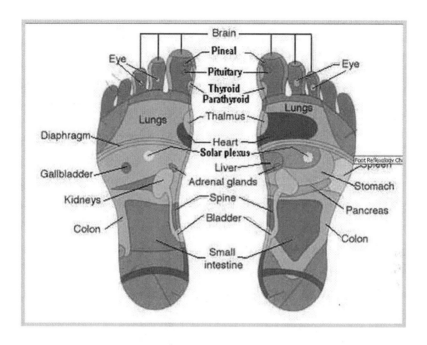

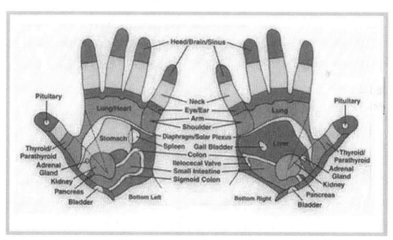

- *Auricular Therapy:* Similar to acupuncture, acupressure, or reflexology, auricular therapy stimulates small reflex points on and around the ears by massaging the essential oil into the area. (Try some Lavender to help calm an upset child.)

- *Hot or Cold Compresses:* Soak a cloth or towel in cool water with drops of your favorite essential oil to place over the area of concern.

Or wrap the cloth/towel in a hot water bottle to use as a warm compress. (A muscle and joint blend and a cool or warm compress on the muscles is amazing.)

- *Bathing, Foot Baths, Etc.:* You can add essential oils to your bathwater, to your bath salts, or to a foot bath to soak in. (Melaleuca in a foot bath helps soothe itchy feet.) When using it in these ways, it's often a good idea to mix with a carrier oil to help disperse the oil and protect your skin from getting multiple drops all in one (potentially very sensitive) area!

- *Personal Care:* You can use essential oils as a natural deodorant (applied "neat", diluted, or in a homemade deodorant recipe, depending on your needs and the oil in question), as part of a skin care regimen, added to lotion or moisturizers, and so on. (An anti-aging blend might be a wonderful oil for skin care, from fine lines to irritated skin.)

Internally

It is important to note that **not all essential oils can be used internally**, nor should all people use them in this way. The *FDA* has listed certain essential oils as *"Generally Recognized as Safe"* for internal use. But they still come with precautions. It is strongly advised to work with a health professional, an aromatherapist, before taking essential oils internally.

There are more precautions for learning how to use essential oils internally than any other application. Remember, essential oils are potent...and the more potent they are, the more you should use them wisely and with education. Even though some oils are generally benign (you could zest a lemon and get more oils than you would normally want to use internally in a day), some require more care. This doesn't mean if you accidentally ingest an oil, that you're going to die. In most cases, you would have to drink a whole bottle (or many bottles) to see any real negative effects. But it is important to keep oils out of the reach of children, especially ones that might smell like food to them.

Some of the most recognized precautions are:

- *Less is More:* Instead of using multiple drops of an oil internally, such as in a veggie capsule, start off with one to see how it works.

- *Increase Frequency before Drops:* Your liver can only tolerate oils in small doses. It's a better idea to use one drop 30-90 minutes apart, rather than 3-4 drops all at once.

- *There's a Time and Place:* Not all needs will respond to internal use. And sometimes topically works just as well (such as digestive oils massaged over the belly). I like to save my internal use for when I really feel I need it.

- *Limit Your Daily Drops:* The general consensus is to consume no more than 10-25 drops of all essential oils per day (25 being for oils such as citruses). You might be able to push this limit with citrus oils, but I stick to the lower end should I ever have a need for a stronger oil. And if you really don't *need* it daily, it's better to save it for when you do.

- *Certain Oils = More Caution:* Oils high in phenols (such as oregano, cinnamon, thyme, etc.) are generally more likely to accumulate in the liver. Use these with care. For a very general guideline/starting point, the hotter the oil, the more precaution. And if you wouldn't normally eat it, think twice before consuming its oil.

- **Dilute:** Even if you're putting your oil in a veggie capsule, while it may not always be necessary, but it's still a good idea to dilute with an edible carrier oil, such as raw coconut oil, olive oil, etc. This helps to ensure less potential irritation to any mucous membranes.

- **Some People Should Just Avoid It:** If you are pregnant, nursing, have a major health concern, a compromised immune system, or liver issues, I would recommend avoiding internal use of most oils until you speak with your naturopathic physician.

If you are using an oil internally, these are possible ways on **how to use essential oils internally:**

- **Cooking:** Many oils, such as Oregano, can be used in cooking or baking. Usually one drop (or less!) is enough, although certain recipes may call for more. Start small at first. Even though something like Oregano is an oil to use internally in moderation, using it in cooking is much safer; you get less than a drop in your meal portion, and some of those properties may be diminished with the heat.

- **Drinking:** Adding Peppermint or Lemon to water is great for helping to support digestion or energy, respectively. For single uses you can add one drop to a minimum 4 oz. of rice milk, almond milk, water, etc. and drink as needed. Remember: **Water and oil don't mix.** Your oil will float to the top and you can get too much at once that way. Mix careful and avoid mixing hot oils with non-oil based liquids for strong oils that may irritate the skin.

- **Supplemental:** Add a drop to 1 tsp of honey to take as a supplement or you can even purchase empty veggie capsules, and add the oils indicated to take daily. (Don't make these in advance as they can dissolve the capsules.) You can also purchase specially formulated essential oil supplements for supporting digestion, energy, immunity, or to supplement your fatty acids, give your children chewables, and more.

- **Vaginal or Rectal Insertion:** These are considered to be more advanced techniques of how to use essential oils, and one to use more caution with. You do *not* want to find out that you're sensitive to an oil this way! Normally the oil is diluted first, and I would recommend working with a naturopath before going this route. For a more beginner's route, you can try diluting first and then adding to a bath instead.

Again, know your brand and use careful consideration with internal application!

Externally

Here are a few extra ideas for **using essential oils around the home**:

- Add 1 drop of a Melaleuca oil to the sink when you're washing dishes.

- Add a few drops of your favorite essential oils to the washing machine, to the wet clothes before they go in the dryer, or misted on fabric before they are dried on a clothes lines.

- Household essential oil uses include oils like Lemon that will remove many stains, and Lime *very* effectively removes gum, stickers, and other residue from most surfaces.

- Many oils have natural antiviral or natural antifungal properties and can be added to natural household cleaners, such as sprays, carpet deodorizers, furniture polish (lemon specifically), and so on. Try mixing your favorite aroma with baking soda for a carpet powder before vacuuming.

- You can even add oils or oil blends to household paint, craft paint or supplies, children's dough, etc. to create a more pleasant aroma. The ratio will vary depending on what you're using it for, anything from 2-3 drops for dough to a whole bottle for a gallon of paint.

- Peppermint or Arborvitae will easily repel ants and many other crawling insects that like to invade the home. Place a few drops on a cotton ball and hide around the entrances of your home, windows, behind the fridge, etc.

- And some insect repelling essential oils are *amazing* for mosquitoes. They can also be used to repel household insects, too.

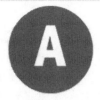 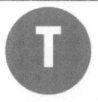 

Aromatically

- Inhale from Bottle
- Inhale from Hands
- Diffuse

Best to ...
- Affect Mood
- Cleans Air
- Ease Breathing

Topically

- Apply directly to skin on area of discomfort
- Rub on bottoms of feet
- Massage

Best to ...
- Immediate Comfort
- Boost Immune System

Internally

- Add to water/juice
- Drop under tongue
- Fill empty gel cap

Best to help...
- Digestive system
- Mouth / Throat
- Liver
- Urogenital tract

SAFETY TIPS FOR ESSENTIAL OIL USAGE

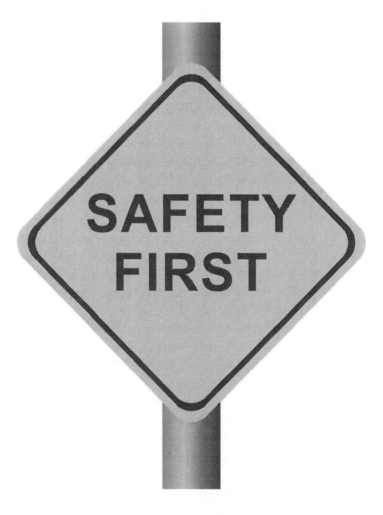

One of the most important things to think about when coming to essential oil use is safety. Safety involves a state of being free from risk or occurrence of injury, harm, or danger.

Factors that influence the safety of essential oils include:

- **Quality of essential oil being utilized** – Adulterated essential oils increase the likelihood of an adverse response and hence the need for pure, authentic, and genuine essential oils is of the utmost importance.

- **Chemical composition of the oil** – Essential oils rich in aldehydes (e.g., citronellal, citral) and phenols (e.g., cinnamic aldehyde, eugenol) may cause reactions. Essential oils rich in these constituents should always be diluted prior to application.

- **Method of application** – Essential oils may be applied topically, inhaled, diffused or taken internally. Each of these methods have safety issues which need to be considered.

- **Dosage/dilution to be applied** – Most aromatherapy oil based blends will be between 1 and 5 percent dilutions, which typically does not represent a safety concern. As one increases dilution, potential reactions may take place depending on the individual essential oil, the area in which the oil is applied, and other factors related to the user's own sensitivity levels.

- **Integrity of area the oil is to be applied** – Damaged, diseased, or inflamed skin is often more permeable to essential oils and may be more sensitive to dermal reactions. It is potentially dangerous to put undiluted essential oils on to damaged, diseased or inflamed skin. Under these circumstances the skin condition may be worsened, and larger amounts of oil than normal will be absorbed. Sensitization reactions are also more likely to occur.

- **Age of patient** – Very young and very old are more sensitive to the potency of essential oils.

Possible Dermal Reactions

Dermal or skin reactions that may occur with essential oils include: irritation, sensitization and phototoxicity/photosensitization.

Dermal irritant – A dermal irritant will produce an immediate effect of irritation on the skin. The reaction will be represented on the skin as blotchy or redness, which may be painful to some individuals. The severity of the reaction will depend on the concentration (dilution) applied. The chart below gives some examples of these:

Essential Oil	Latin Name
Bay	*Pimento racemosa*
Cinnamon bark or leaf	*Cinnamomum zeylanicum**
Clove bud	*Syzygium aromaticum*
Citronella	*Cymbopogon nardus*
Cumin	*Cuminum cyminum*
Lemongrass	*Cymbopogon citratus*
Lemon verbena	*Lippia citriodora*
Oregano	*Origanum vulgare*
Tagetes	*Tagetes minuta*
Thyme ct. thymol	*Thymus vulgaris*

*bark is more irritating than leaf

Dermal sensitization – Dermal sensitization is a type of allergic reaction. It occurs on first exposure to a substance, but on this occasion, the noticeable effect on the skin will be slight or absent. However, subsequent exposure to the same material, or to a similar one with which there is cross-sensitization, produces a severe inflammatory reaction brought about by cells of the immune system (T-lymphocytes). The reaction will be represented on the skin as blotchy or redness, which may be painful to some individuals.

The problem with dermal sensitization is that once it occurs with a specific essential oil the individual is most likely going to be sensitive to it for many years and perhaps for the remainder of his/her life. The best way to prevent sensitization is to avoid known dermal sensitizers and avoid applying the same essential oils every day for lengthy periods of time. Sensitization is, to an extent, unpredictable, as some individuals will be sensitive to a potential allergen and some will not.

Essential Oil	Latin Name
Cassia	*Cinnamomum cassia*
Cinnamon bark	*Cinnamomum zeylanicum*
Peru balsam	*Myroxylon pereirae*
Verbena absolute	*Lippia citriodora*
Tea absolute	*Camellia sinensis*
Turpentine oil	*Pinus spp.*
Backhousia	*Backhousia citriodora*
Inula	*Inula graveolens*
Oxidized oils from Pinaceae family (e.g., Pinus and Cupressus species) and Rutaceae family (e.g., citrus oils)	

Photosensitization – An essential oil that exhibits this quality will cause burning or skin pigmentation changes, such as tanning, on exposure to sun or similar light (ultraviolet rays). Reactions can range from a mild color change through to deep weeping burns. Do not use or recommend the use of photosensitizing essential oils prior to going into a sun tanning booth or the sun. Recommend that the client stay out of the sun or sun tanning booth for at least twenty-four hours after treatment if photosensitizing essential oils were applied to the skin. Certain drugs, such as tetracycline, increase the photosensitivity of the skin, thus increasing the harmful effects of photosensitizing essential oils under the necessary conditions.

Essential Oil	Latin Name
Angelica root	*Angelica archangelica*
Bergamot	*Citrus bergamia*
Cumin	*Cuminum cyminum*
Distilled or expressed grapefruit (low risk)	*Citrus paradisi*
Expressed lemon	*Citrus limon*
Expressed lime	*Citrus medica*
Orange, bitter (expressed)	*Citrus aurantium*
Rue	*Ruta graveolens*

The table below includes a list of non-phototoxic citrus oils:

Essential Oil	Latin Name
Bergamot: Bergapteneless (FCF: Furanocoumarin Free)	*Citrus bergamia*
Distilled lemon	*Citrus limon*
Distilled lime	*Citrus medica*
Mandarin – Tangerine	*Citrus reticulata*
Sweet orange	*Citrus sinensis*
Expressed tangerine	*Citrus reticulata*
Yuzu oil (expressed or distilled)	*Citrus juno*

Idiosyncratic irritation or sensitization – Idiosyncratic irritation or sensitization is an uncharacteristic or unusual reaction to a commonly used essential oil. This type of reaction is difficult to predict and rarely occurs but is a possibility.

Mucous membrane irritant – A mucous membrane irritant will produce a heating or drying effect on the mucous membranes of the mouth, eyes, nose, and reproductive organs. It is recommended that mucus membrane irritating essential oils not be used in a full body bath unless placed in a dispersant first (e.g., milk, vegetable oil). It would also be wise to put the dispersed essential oils into the water after you have gotten into the bath. Bay, clove, cinnamon bark, lemongrass, and thyme ct. thymol essential oils should be avoided in baths completely.

Essential Oil	Latin Name
Bay	*Pimento racemosa*
Caraway	*Carum carvi*
Cinnamon bark or leaf	*Cinnamomum zeylanicum*
Clove bud or leaf	*Syzygium aromaticum*
Lemongrass	*Cymbopogon citratus*
Peppermint	*Mentha x piperita*
Thyme ct. thymol	*Thymus vulgaris*

Other Safety Considerations

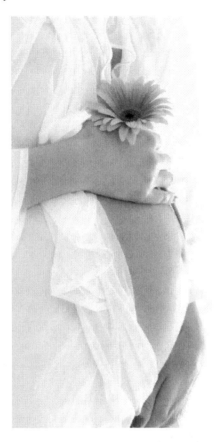

Pregnancy – The use of essential oils during pregnancy is a controversial topic and one that is yet to be fully understood. The main concern during pregnancy appears to be the risk of essential oil constituents crossing over into the placenta. Many researchers believe that crossing the placenta does not necessarily mean that there is a risk of toxicity to the fetus; this will depend on the toxicity and the plasma concentration of the compound. It is probable that essential oil metabolites cross the placenta due to the intimate (but not direct) contact between maternal and embryonic or fetal blood.

Essential oils that appear to be safe include cardamon, German and Roman chamomile, frankincense, geranium, ginger, neroli, patchouli, petitgrain, rosewood, rose, sandalwood, and other nontoxic essential oils. It would also be prudent to avoid the internal or undiluted application of essential oils throughout pregnancy.

Essential oils to Avoid throughout Pregnancy, Labor, and while Breastfeeding:

Essential Oil	Latin Name
Aniseed	*Pimpinella anisum*
Angelica	*Angelica arhangelica*
Basil ct. estragole	*Ocimum basilicum*
Birch	*Betula lenta*
Black Pepper	*Piper nigrum*
Camphor	*Cinnamomum camphora*
Cinnamon	*Cinnamomum verum, Cinnamomum zeylanicum*
Chamomile	*Chamaemelum nobile, Chamaemelum matricaria*
Clary Sage	*Salvia sclarea*
Clove	*Syzygium aromaticum*
Fennel	*Foeniculum vulgare*
Fir	*Abies alba, abies balsamea, abies grandis*
Ginger	*Zingiber officinale*
Horseradish	*Armoracia lapathifolia gilib*
Hyssop	*Hyssopus officinalis*
Jasmine	*Jasminum officinalis*
Juniper	*Juniperus Communis*
Marjoram	*Origanum majorana*
Mugwort	*Artemisia vulgaris*

Mustard	*Brassica nigra, Brassica hirta*
Myrrh	*Commiphora myrrha*
Nutmeg	*Myristica fragrans*
Oregano	*Origanum vulgare*
Parsley seed or leaf	*Petroselinum sativum*
Pennyroyal	*Mentha pulegium*
Peppermint	*Mentha x Piperita*
Rosemary	*Rosmarinus officinalis*
Sage	*Salvia officinalis*
Tansy	*Tanacetum vulgare*
Tarragon	*Artemisia dracunculus*
Thuja	*Thuja occidentalis*
Thyme	*Thymus vulgaris*
Wintergreen	*Gaultheria procumbens*
Wormwood	*Artemisia absinthium*

Eye Safety – When using essential oils, you must be careful with your eyes. The following tips are considered the most important:

- Undiluted essential oils should not be applied to the eyes.

- It is rash to suggest that essential oils are commonly used to treat eye problems

- Eye injuries and diseases are medical conditions, and any product claiming to treat them is a medicine, subject to drug legislation.

- There is currently no evidence that applying dilutions of essential oil to the eyes will be beneficial in any condition.

- Diluted (5%) tea tree oil may help eradicate eyelash mites, but it should not be placed into the eyes.

General Safety Precautions

1. Keep all essential oils stored out of reach of children and pets.

2. Do not use or recommend the use of photosensitizing essential oils prior to going into the sun. Keep out of the sun for at least twenty-four hours after treatment if photosensitizing essential oils were applied.

3. Avoid prolonged use of the same essential oils.

4. Avoid the use of essential oils you know nothing about. Research and get to know the oil prior to using it.

5. Avoid the use of undiluted essential oils, unless otherwise indicated.

6. If you suspect that you may be sensitive to specific essential oils or if you have known allergies or sensitivities, it may be wise to perform a patch test.

7. Know the safety data on each essential oil and place into context of use and knowledge.

8. Use caution if you are, or trying to become pregnant.

9. Keep essential oils away from the eyes.

10. Essential oils are highly flammable substances and should be kept away from direct contact with flames, such as candles, fire, matches, cigarettes, and gas cookers.

11. Make sure your treatment room has good ventilation.

12. Do not use essential oils internally unless properly trained in the safety issues of doing so.

Safety Measures

- If essential oil droplets accidentally get into the eye (or eyes) a cotton cloth or similar should be imbued with a fatty oil, such as olive or sesame, and carefully swiped over the closed lid. And / Or, immediately flush the eyes with cool water.

- If an essential oil causes dermal irritation, apply a small amount of vegetable oil or cream to the area affected and discontinue use of essential oil or product that has caused dermal irritation.

- If a child appears to have drunk several spoonfuls of essential oil, contact the nearest poison control unit (often listed in the front of a telephone directory). Keep the bottle for identification and encourage the child to drink whole or 2% milk. Do not try to induce vomiting.

ALL YOU NEED TO
KNOW ABOUT ALLERGIES

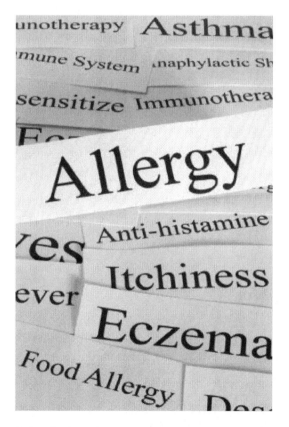

An allergy is defined as "*a damaging immune response by the body to a substance, especially a particular food, pollen, fur, or dust, to which it has become hypersensitive*". Any substance that triggers an allergic reaction is called an **allergen**.

Some of the most common allergens include:

- grass and tree pollen (hay fever)

- dust mites

- animal dander (tiny flakes of skin or hair)

- food products (particularly fruits, shellfish and nuts)

An allergy develops when the body's immune system reacts to an allergen as though it is a threat, like an infection. It produces antibodies to fight off the allergen, in a reaction called the *"immune response"*.

The next time a person comes into contact with the allergen, the body "re-members" the previous exposure and produces more of the antibodies. This causes the release of chemicals in the body that lead to an allergic reaction.

Symptoms of an allergy can include:

- Sneezing

- Wheezing

- Itchy eyes

- Skin rashes

- Swelling.

The nature of the symptoms depends on the allergen. For example, you may experience problems with your airways if you breathe in pollen.

There are considered to be **three categories of allergy**, and listed below is how these allergies can develop:

- *Allergy* – this is a reaction produced by the body's immune system when it encounters a normally harmless substance.

- *Sensitivity* – this is the exaggeration of a normal side effect produced by contact with a substance. For example, the caffeine in a cup of coffee may cause extreme symptoms, such as palpitations and trembling, when it would usually only have this effect when taken in much larger doses.

- *Intolerance* – this is where a substance (such as lactose) causes unpleasant symptoms (such as diarrhea) for a variety of reasons, but does not involve the immune system. People with an intolerance to certain foods can typically eat a small amount without having any problems. In contrast, people with a food allergy will have a bad reaction even if they come into contact with a tiny amount of the food to which they are allergic.

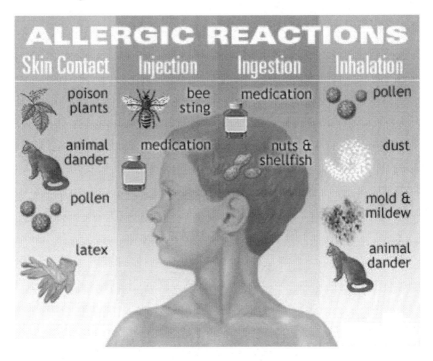

Now, you may be aware that allergies are quite common – it seems that everyone knows someone who is allergic to *something* – but, did you know that according to data collected by the *National Institution of Health*, **more than 50% of Americans suffer from one or more allergies?** That's a *lot* of people!

4 Most Common Allergy Types

Here is a list of **the most common allergies** that people suffer from:

1. Food Allergies

- *Milk Allergy* – If you suffer from a milk allergy, strictly avoiding milk and food containing milk and milk products is the only way to prevent a reaction, which can include immediate wheezing, vomiting, and hives.

- *Egg Allergy* – Egg allergies – especially to egg whites – are more common in children than in adults and reactions range from mild to severe.

- *Wheat Allergy* – If you are allergic to any wheat protein strictly avoiding wheat and wheat products is the only way to prevent a reaction, which can include stomach upset, eczema, allergic rhinitis, bronchospasm (asthma-like symptoms) and even anaphylaxis.

- *Nut (Peanut) Allergy* – If you suffer from a nut allergy, strictly avoiding nuts, including peanuts and tree nuts like cashews and walnuts, and food containing nuts is the only way to prevent a reaction.

- *Fish Allergy* – If your doctor is able to identify exactly which type of fish causes your allergies, then you only need to eliminate that species of fish from your diet. For the majority of fish allergy sufferers, this is not an option and all fish must be avoided.

- *Shellfish Allergy* – If you are allergic to shellfish, you need to keep away from seafood – even when it's cooking as that can spark a reaction.

- *Sulfite Allergy* – Sulfites are a group of sulfur-based compounds that may occur naturally or may be added to food as an enhancer and preservative. The FDA estimates that one out of 100 people is sensitive to the compounds.

- *Soy Allergy* – Soy allergies start with soybeans. Soybeans are legumes. Other foods in the legume family include navy beans, kidney beans, string beans, black beans, pinto beans, chickpeas (garbanzo or chichi beans), lentils, carob, licorice, and peanuts.

- *Casein Allergy* – If a glass of milk or a slice of pizza causes swollen lips, hives, or other significant symptoms, you may have an allergy to casein, a protein in milk.

2. <u>Seasonal Allergies</u>

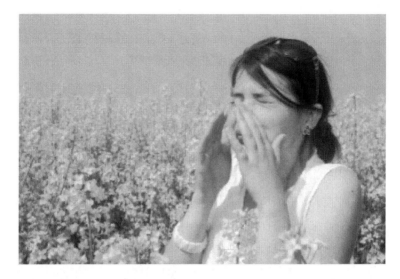

- *Spring Allergies* – Spring is the time of year that we normally think of when it comes to seasonal allergies. As the trees start to bloom and the pollen gets airborne, allergy sufferers begin their annual ritual of sniffling and sneezing. Trees and grass are the worst spring triggers.

- *Summer Allergies* – Although spring most readily comes to mind when we think of allergies, many of the same allergic triggers that can make us miserable in the spring persist into summer. Weeds, grasses and insects are the main summer triggers.

- *Fall Allergies* – The allergy triggers might be slightly different, but they can be just as misery-inducing as the flower pollen that fills the air in the spring and summer. Pollen, fruits, vegetables and dust mites are the main fall triggers.

- *Winter Allergies* – Dust mites, molds and animals are the biggest trigger of winter allergies. The symptoms can be coughing, watery eyes and runny nose.

3. Pet Allergies

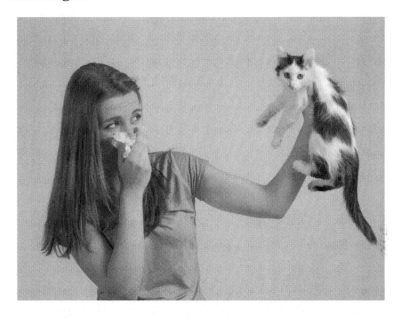

- *Dog Allergy* – For a person with dog allergies, life in a dog-loving country isn't easy. Nearly 40% of U.S. households have a dog. Dog dander gets everywhere, including places where dogs have never set a paw.

- *Cat Allergy* – About 10% of the U.S. population has pet allergies and cats are among the most common culprits. Cat allergies are twice as common as dog allergies. But contrary to what you might think, it's not the fur or hair that's the real problem. People with cat allergies are really allergic to proteins in the cat's saliva, urine, and dander (dried flakes of skin).

4. <u>Other Allergies</u>

- *Hay Fever* – Hay fever is an immune disorder characterized by an allergic response to pollen grains and other substances. Also known as allergic rhinitis, there are two types: seasonal, which occurs only during the time of year in which certain plants pollinate, and perennial, which occurs all year round.

- *Allergic Conjunctivitis (Pink Eye)* – Pink eye caused by bacteria, viruses, or STDs can spread easily from person to person but is not a serious health risk if diagnosed promptly; allergic conjunctivitis is not contagious.

- *Hives (Urticaria)* – Hives, also known as urticaria, are an outbreak of swollen, pale red bumps, patches, or welts on the skin that appear suddenly – either as a result of allergies, or for other reasons.

- *Allergies to Poison Ivy, Oak, and Sumac* – Poison ivy, poison oak, and poison sumac are plants that contain an irritating, oily sap called urushiol. Urushiol triggers an allergic reaction when it comes into contact with skin, resulting in an itchy rash, which can appear within hours of exposure or up to several days later.

- *Allergies to Insect Stings (Bee Stings)* – Bee, wasp, yellow jacket, hornet, or fire ant stings are the insect stings that most often trigger allergies. However, most people are not allergic to insect stings and may mistake a normal sting reaction for an allergic reaction.

- *Mold Allergy* – People with mold allergies, however, may have a reaction if exposed to too much of the fungus.

- *Pollen Allergies* – For most people, a change of seasons signals the beginning of long, lazy days or cool, crisp evenings. But for the one in 10 Americans who suffers from pollen allergies, changing seasons can mean misery.

- *Sun Reactions of the Skin* – Most people's skin will burn if there is enough exposure to ultraviolet radiation. However, some people burn particularly easily or develop exaggerated skin reactions to sunlight.

- *Aspirin Allergy (Salicylate Allergy)* – Salicylates are chemicals found naturally in plants and are a major ingredient of aspirin and other pain-relieving medications. They are also found in many fruits and vegetables as well as in many common health and beauty products.

- *Cosmetic Allergy* – Although cosmetics can help us feel more beautiful, they can cause skin irritation or allergic reactions. Certain ingredients used in cosmetics, such as fragrances and preservatives, can act as allergens, substances that trigger an allergic reaction.

- *Nickel Allergy* – A nickel allergy is a skin reaction that develops after exposure to nickel or items containing the metal.

- *Drug Allergy* – Many drugs can cause adverse side effects, and certain medicines can trigger allergic reactions. In an allergic reaction, the immune system mistakenly responds to a drug by creating an immune response against it.

- *Dust Allergy* – Life with dust allergies – whether they're yours or a family member's – comes with a load of questions. For instance, might a dust allergy explain your child's never-ending cold symptoms?

- *Chemical Allergy* – They promise to make your skin soft, your hair shiny, and your laundry springtime fresh, but for some people the chemicals in shampoos, cosmetics, and detergents trigger allergic skin reactions.

- *Penicillin Allergy* – A penicillin allergy is an allergic reaction that occurs when your body's immune system overreacts to penicillin antibiotics.

The Frightening Statistics

Below are six different visual aids from *Centers for Disease Control and Prevention* (www.cdc.gov) which demonstrate just how many people are affected by allergies. This should give you a better idea of just *why* it's so important to look at them, and why finding an alternative treatment is *so* important.

Figure 1. Percentage of children under age 18 years who had a reported food or digestive allergy in the past 12 months, by age, sex, and race and ethnicity group: United States, 2007

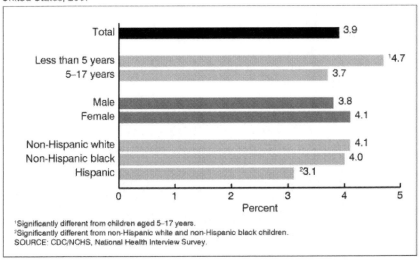

Figure 1. Percentage of children aged 0–17 years with a reported allergic condition in the past 12 months: United States, 1997–2011

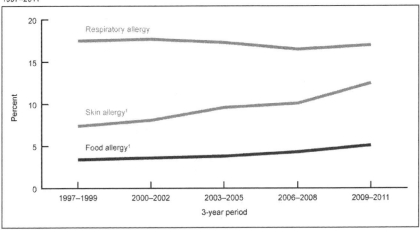

WHEAT FREE

15 MILLION AMERICANS HAVE FOOD ALLERGIES.

6 MILLION, OR **8%**, OF CHILDREN.

GLUTEN FREE

200,000 ANNUAL **ER** VISITS FROM ALLERGIC REACTIONS OCCUR ANNUALLY.

DAIRY FREE

2,000 HOSPITALIZATIONS FROM ALLERGIC REACTIONS ANNUALLY.

150 FOOD ALLERGEN-RELATED DEATHS ANNUALLY.

LACTOSE FREE

50% OF FOOD ALLERGY RELATED DEATHS OCCUR AWAY FROM HOME.

NUT FREE

AN ESTIMATED **20%** OF FOOD ALLERGIC INDIVIDUALS REQUIRE SOME TYPE OF DIETARY ACCOMMODATION FOR AVOIDANCE.

SUGAR FREE

STUDIES INDICATE AN **18%** INCREASE IN PERSONS WITH FOOD ALLERGIES FROM **1997 – 2007.**

SHELLFISH FREE

EGG FREE

6 PROVEN WAYS TO DIAGNOSE ALLERGIES

If you suspect that you have allergies, the first thing that you'll want to do is get a second opinion from a medical expert.

These are the tests that doctors will do to **test for allergies**:

- **Skin prick testing –** Skin prick testing is mainly used to investigate allergies to:

  - airborne allergens

  - certain foods

  - insect venoms

  - certain drug allergies.

  The test involves putting a drop of liquid allergen onto your forearm, followed by a gentle pin prick through the drop. If you are allergic to the substance, an itchy, red bump will appear within 15 minutes. Skin prick testing is very safe and can be performed in people of all ages. Antihistamines interfere with the results, so they need to be stopped for several days before the test.

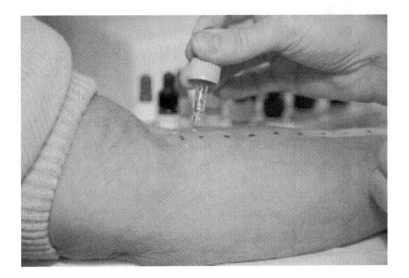

- **Intradermal testing** – Intradermal testing involves injecting a watered-down allergen into the top layer of skin with a very fine needle. It is slightly more painful than the skin prick test and presents a slightly higher risk of an allergic reaction, but is still very safe. Intradermal testing is usually used to investigate allergies to certain medications or insect venom.

- **Blood tests** – Blood tests may be used instead of, or alongside, skin prick tests to help diagnose common allergies. The tests used are known as specific IgE tests or radioallergosorbent tests (RASTs).

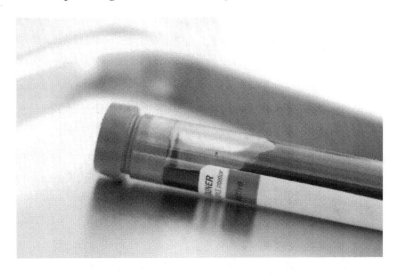

- **Patch tests** – Patch tests are used to investigate a type of eczema known as contact dermatitis. A small amount of the suspected allergen is added to special metal discs, which are then taped to your skin for 48 hours and monitored for a reaction. This test is usually carried out at a dermatology (skin) department in a hospital.

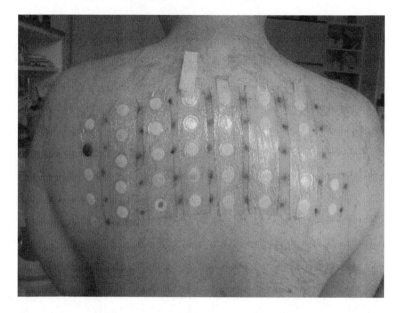

- **Challenge testing** – A food challenge may be used to diagnose a food allergy if skin and blood tests have not given a clear diagnosis. During the test, you're given the food you think you are allergic to in gradually increasing amounts, to see how you react under close supervision. This test is riskier than other forms of testing, but is the most accurate way to diagnose food and certain medication allergies.

- **Allergy testing kits** – The use of commercial allergy-testing kits is not recommended. These tests are often of a lower standard than those provided by the accredited clinics. Allergy tests should be interpreted by a qualified professional who has detailed knowledge of your symptoms and medical history.

TRADITIONAL ALLERGY TREATMENTS

Here are the most commonly used traditional allergy treatments:

- **Antihistamines** – When your body comes into contact with whatever your allergic trigger is – pollen, ragweed, pet dander, dust mites, for example – it makes chemicals called *histamines*. They cause the tissue in your nose to swell (making it stuffy), your nose and eyes to run, and your eyes, nose and sometimes mouth to itch. Sometimes you may also get an itchy rash on your skin, called *hives*. Antihistamines reduce or block histamines, so they stop allergy symptoms.

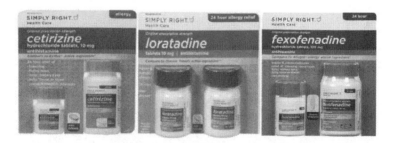

- **Decongestants** – Allergies make the lining of your nose swell. Decongestants shrink swollen blood vessels and tissues. That relieves the congestion. But decongestants can't help with sneezing or itching. Decongestants come in pills, liquids, nose drops, and nasal sprays.

- **Anticholinergic Nasal Allergy Sprays** – When sprayed into each nostril, anticholinergic nasal sprays decrease secretions from the glands lining the nasal passage. This diminishes the symptom of runny nose.

- **Steroid Nasal Sprays** – These drugs decrease inflammation within the nasal passages, thereby relieving nasal symptoms.

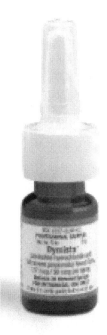

- **Allergy Eye Drops** – Allergy eye drops are liquid medicines used to treat symptoms of eye allergies. Eye allergy symptoms include burning of the eye, feeling like something is in the eye, itchy eyes, red (bloodshot) eyes, swelling of the eyelid and tearing.

- **Leukotriene Inhibitors** – *Montelukast (Singulair)* is a drug that relieves allergy symptoms and is also used to prevent asthma attacks. It reduces congestion in your nose and also cuts down on sneezing, itching, and eye allergies. For people with allergies and asthma, it helps reduce inflammation in your airways. It works by stopping the action of a chemical called leukotriene, which causes your nasal passages to swell and make a lot of mucus. The same chemical is also responsible for tightening airways when you have asthma, making it harder to breathe.

- **Mast Cell Inhibitors** – *Cromolyn sodium (Nasalcrom, Crolom),* a mast cell inhibitor, is used to prevent allergic symptoms like runny nose or itchy eyes. Cromolyn sodium must be started 1-2 weeks before pollen season and continued daily to prevent seasonal allergy symptoms. The response is not as strong as that of corticosteroid nasal sprays. These drugs prevent the release of histamine and other chemicals that cause allergic symptoms from mast cells when an individual comes into contact with an allergen like pollen.

- **Allergy Shots** – Allergy shots help your body get used to allergens, the things that trigger an allergic reaction. They don't cure allergies, but eventually your symptoms will get better and you may not have allergic reactions as often. Allergy shots, also called *"immunotherapy"* may work for you if allergy drugs don't work well or you have symptoms more than three months a year.

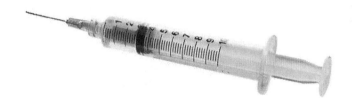

- **Skin Allergies** – The best treatment is *prevention*. Find out what causes your rash and avoid it. You may need to wear gloves to protect your skin. When you have a reaction, try to ease the symptoms and prevent an infection. Don't scratch, even though that's a hard urge to resist. Over-the-counter products and home remedies can help relieve the itching and stop the swelling.

- **Dehumidifiers** – Dust mites are the most common trigger of allergy and asthma symptoms, and they thrive in high humidity. They can live in bedding, curtains, and rugs, as well as the air in your home. A dehumidifier brings down the level of moisture in your home, making it unfriendly to dust mites and limiting the growth of mold and mildew.

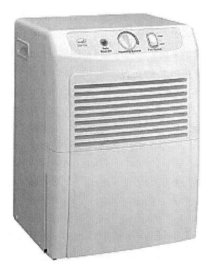

- **Auto-Injector –** An allergy attack can quickly become intense, sometimes leading to *anaphylaxis* – a severe, often life-threatening reaction.
An auto-injector, such as EpiPen, Twinject, or Auvi-Q, can treat extreme allergic reactions with an early, life-saving dose of epinephrine.
Epinephrine is adrenaline, a hormone your body naturally produces.
Among other things, it can help improve breathing, raise blood pressure that's dropping, and reduce swelling.

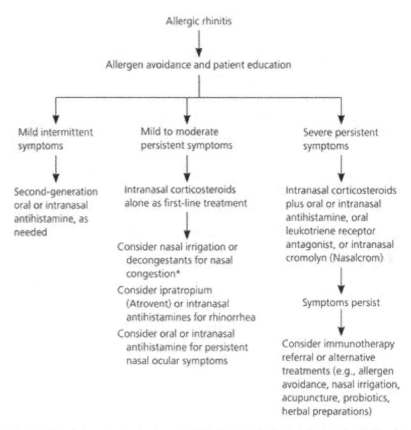

Allergic rhinitis

↓

Allergen avoidance and patient education

Mild intermittent symptoms

↓

Second-generation oral or intranasal antihistamine, as needed

Mild to moderate persistent symptoms

↓

Intranasal corticosteroids alone as first-line treatment

↓

Consider nasal irrigation or decongestants for nasal congestion*

Consider ipratropium (Atrovent) or intranasal antihistamines for rhinorrhea

Consider oral or intranasal antihistamine for persistent nasal ocular symptoms

Severe persistent symptoms

↓

Intranasal corticosteroids plus oral or intranasal antihistamine, oral leukotriene receptor antagonist, or intranasal cromolyn (Nasalcrom)

↓

Symptoms persist

↓

Consider immunotherapy referral or alternative treatments (e.g., allergen avoidance, nasal irrigation, acupuncture, probiotics, herbal preparations)

*—Use of nasal decongestants for longer than three days is cautioned because of risk of rebound congestion.

Top Reasons Why
Traditional Medication Fails

Sometimes this tradition medication doesn't work – which is one of the main reasons people look for alternatives, such as essential oils. Below are the top reasons why this happens:

- **Cutting Corners** – Non-adherence, or not doing all that you can to prevent allergies, is one of the main reasons people continue to suffer.

- **Medication Mistakes** – Forgetting to take the medication you have been prescribed, or not taking it exactly as the instructions direct can cause all sorts of issues.

- **Botched Diagnosis** – If your diagnosis is wrong, your treatment won't be right either. Many people who self-diagnose have this issue.

- **Physical Issues** – Treatments aren't one-size-fits-all, and other issues such as high blood pressure can affect medications.

There is also another reason why people don't like the medication that they're prescribed, why they are eager to try something else and that is the *side effects*. The following are possible reactions to using traditional medicine to help with your allergies:

- An Increase in the Thickness of Lung Secretions

- Drowsiness

- Blood Disorder

- Extra Heartbeat

- Hallucination

- Reaction due to an Allergy

- Seizures

- Blurred Vision

- Confused

- Difficult or Painful Urination

- Dizzy

- Dry Mouth

- Dryness of the Nose

- Excessive Sweating

- Fast Heartbeat

- Head Pain

- Hives

- Involuntary Quivering

- Itching

- Loss of Appetite

- Nervous

- Nightmares

- Over Excitement

- Problems with Eyesight

- Rash

- Ringing in the Ears

- Stomach Cramps

- Sun-Sensitive Skin

- Throat Dryness

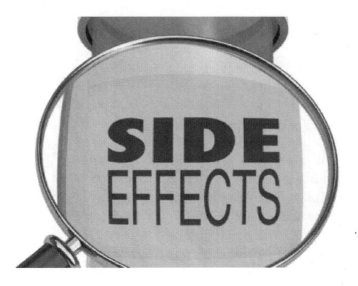

On top of these commonly known side effects, some sources, gives examples of other surprising side effects discovered through their own research:

- Low Libido

- Increased Appetite

- Altered Taste and Smell

- Long Term Health Issues

- Infertility in Women

- Anxiety

- Impairment of Thinking

- Depression

After looking at this list, it's very **easy to see why people are looking for alternatives**. For some people, the side effects of the medication can be worse than the effects of the allergy! If this is the case, it's certainly worth looking elsewhere. Particularly as stress can be one of the surprising triggers of allergies – so worrying about what you're taking can have negative effects in more than one way.

ALLERGY TREATMENT WITH ESSENTIAL OILS

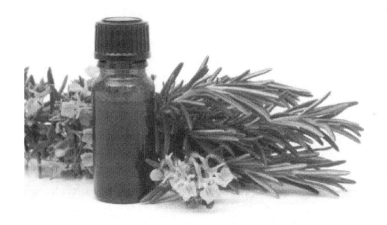

So now that we've looked at the reasons people are turning away from traditional medication for treating their allergies, it's time to examine *why* essential oils is not only a better option, but it's the most effective way to treat allergies.

Benefits

According to most sources, the **Top benefits** for choosing essential oils are:

- They are **easy** (and fun) to use, and work!

- They are **non-toxic** to our body, our kids and our pets (only if used correctly). Not oils are safe for children, and also be careful with using essential oils for cats.

- They are friendly to our **environment** and the planet.

- They promote emotional and physical **well-being**.

- They improve the **quality** of our lives.

- They give us an **alternative solution**.

- They have more **benefits** than side effects.

In particular, when it comes to allergies, traditional medication can have more of a negative impact on your health, with very little help. Another issue suffers often come across is **tolerance**. They become so used to their medication, that it no longer works as effectively. This is when we need to start looking at something new.

What you might not know about essential oils is that they can actually heal you at a cellular level. This means the level of help that they can give you when it comes to your allergies is phenomenal.

Side Effects Of Essential Oils

Now, you may know that essential oils work differently to traditional medicine, but you might not know *why* or why they aren't included in the same field.

Essential oils are wholly natural and cannot be patented; which means that you'll never see an essential oil in a pharmaceutical drug. As such, you can expect that the vast majority of mainstream healthcare practitioners will never recommend essential oils as therapeutic alternatives to drugs. More importantly, because essential oils cannot be patented, drug companies will not waste money studying them. This limits our scientific knowledge of essential oils greatly, and the majority of what we know about them are things that have been passed down through thousands of years of personal use and experimentation.

Despite the fact that these oils are wholly natural, they still carry a **risk of side effects**. Even though the side effects of essential oils are nothing compared to what you will get from traditional medicine, there are some things to look out for. After all, it's better to be safe than sorry!

The following are side effects to look out for:

- **Skin Discoloration** – Some essential oils can cause you to burn in the sunlight. Before you head out to the beach or to a tanning booth, make sure you don't have photosensitizing oil on your skin. Reactions can range from discoloration to oozing burns. Did your friend selling oils mention that? Photosensitizing oils include, but aren't limited to Bergamot, Lemon, Lime and Cumin.

- **Pregnancy Complications** – Babies, pregnant women and breast-feeding women should use extreme caution. When dealing with babies, kids, pregnant women and breastfeeding women, oils should be heavily diluted – such as one percent of essential oil in a safe carrier oil, like coconut oil. Rosemary and spike lavender should never be used on pregnant women, even diluted. Don't use oils at all on babies under one year of age. Your safest bet is to stick to products made specifically for babies and pregnant women instead of making something on your own or using undiluted oils. The National Association for Holistic Aromatherapy recommends that pregnant women avoid the following oils, among others; Sage, Mugwort, Tarragon and Wintergreen essential oil.

- **Skin Irritation** – A drop of peppermint oil on the back of your neck can help a headache – or it can cause serious skin irritation. Many oils irritate the skin when applied undiluted. Do a small spot test before applying oils to your skin, even when they're diluted in a moisturizing carrier oil. Don't assume that every oil is safe to apply directly to your skin. These are just a few oils that can cause skin irritation; Lemongrass, Cinnamon, Citronella and Bay.

- **Danger to Very Small Pets** – Essential oils aren't safe for pets. Unless you own a very large animal, like a horse, don't try using essential oils on your pets. Only use essential oil products under the supervision of your vet.

- **Danger to Pre-existing Illnesses** – Even inhaling some oils can cause side effects for people with health problems. Don't use oils on people with preexisting conditions like asthma or heart problems unless you're working with a trained aromatherapist. Aromatherapy training involves 200 or more hours of classes, and includes studying chemistry and drug interactions. Don't take your friend's word for it just because she's selling oils.

- **Death or Illness when Swallowed** – Really hardcore essential oil enthusiasts take oils orally. This isn't something an everyday essential oil fan should try. Oils like pennyroyal and wintergreen can be fatal if swallowed. Some toxic oils can cause miscarriage when swallowed. Others can become highly irritating when they've been kept on the shelf too long. Skip oral use unless you're using oils under the supervision of a medical professional.

These scenarios are very extreme, but reconfirm that you should always consult a health professional before taking any products. Remember that they are a medication, and should be treated as such.

Essential Oils and Pharmaceuticals Compared

Essential Oils	Pharmaceuticals
Properties	Properties
1. Natural, wildcrafted or grown organically	1. Unnatural, synthetic chemically or genetically engineered
2. Hundreds of constituents, not all known	2. One or two active ingredients, all of which are known
3. Never two batches the same.	3. Every batch the same (Purity)
4. Not patentable (God made)	4. Patentable (man made)
Effects and Consequences	Effects and Consequences
5. Restores natural function	5. Inhibits natural function
6. No adverse interactions	6. Many adverse interactions
7. Antiviral	7. Usually not antiviral
8. Improves intercellular communication	8. Disrupts intercellular communication
9. Corrects and restores proper cellular memory (DNA)	9. Garbles and confuses cellular memory (DNA)
10. Cleanses receptor sites	10. Blocks receptor sites
11. Builds the immune system	11. Depresses immune system
12. Emotionally balancing	12. Emotionally unbalancing
13. Side effects beneficial	13. Side effects harmful
14. Leads toward independence and wellness	14. Leads toward dependence and chronic disease
Philosophy/Paradigm	Philosophy/Paradigm
15. Assumes wellness as natural state, invulnerable to illness	15. Assumes natural state prone and vulnerable to illness
16. Assumes body and mind capable of self-healing	16. Assumes body and mind need external assistance to heal
17. Integrated wholistically, body, mind, and soul as a unit	17. Fragmented, treats body parts, mind and emotions separate
18. Build natural defenses and let body deal with disease	18. Supplant natural defenses and attack disease itself
19. Treats internally at level of cellular intelligence	19. Treats externally at level of gross symptoms
20. Theistic, historic roots in religion when healers were priests	20. Secular, historic roots in materialism motivated by money

Top 5 Essential Oils
To Overcome Allergies

There are a number of essential oils that are perfect for helping with allergies – all of which we will examine in detail in the next chapter, to ensure that you're fully informed. Just to give you an idea, here are most common recommendations:

1. **Lavender** works as a natural antihistamine and possess strong anti-inflammatory properties to treat and relief most allergic reactions. Works great to treat skin rashes or headaches. And not only will it ease your allergic reaction, it has a calming and relaxing effect on body and mind, and smells great.

2. **Peppermint** has a strong, fresh, and minty aroma that works wonders to treat allergic reactions. Especially those that cause respiratory or digestive issues. It has pain-relieving, soothing, cooling, and has anti-inflammatory properties. It helps to open the airways, improves breathing and eases congestion.

3. **Lemon** works as a natural antihistamine, relieves excess mucus, and cools down the inflammation which is the result of an allergic reaction. Lemon essential oil works best in combination with lavender and peppermint.

4. **Eucalyptus** supports the respiratory system and is well known to ease seasonal allergies and asthma attacks.

5. **Roman Chamomile** works wonders to treat rashes, eczema, and other skin condition caused by allergic reaction.

But it's very important to note one ***very powerful* combination** that has been created and is believed to keep allergies away long term. ***Lemon, Lavender*** and ***Peppermint*** make a highly successful blend, perfect for allergy sufferers.

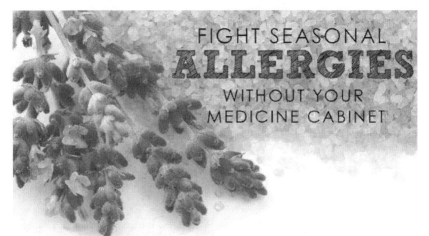

LAVENDER, LEMON AND PEPPERMINT ESSENTIAL
OILS CREATE POWERFUL, ALL-NATURAL ALLERGY RELIEF.

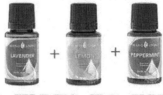

3 WAYS TO USE

1. Add 3 drops of each and rub behind ears and on back of neck.

2. Add 5 drops each to an empty vegetable capsule (available at health food store or Young Living)*

3. Add 1 drop each to a spoonful of local honey for children. For adults you can do 2-3 drops each.*

Lavender, Lemon and Peppermint essential oils can create a powerful all-natural antihistamine. These three oils together can cool down body inflammation resulting from the body's allergic response. Once you combine those 3 oils, they begin to work their magic and you have a wonderful substitution to those synthetic drugs that your body doesn't like to process.

3 ways to use this blend:

1. Add 3 drops each to shot glass of juice or water, swish 10-20 seconds in the mouth and swallow.

2. Add 3 drops each to an empty veggie capsule (available at health food stores).

3. Add 1 drop each to a spoonful of local honey for children or apply to the bottoms of their feet. For adults you can do 2-3 drops each.

(Only take internally if your oils are Certified Pure Therapeutic Grade Oils and you have spoken to a health professional. If your oils are otherwise, rub on the bottoms of your feet and cover with a sock.)

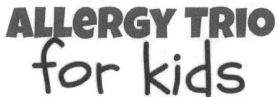

ALLERGY TRIO
for kids

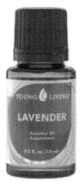
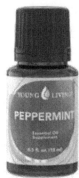
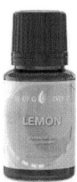

eat one drop of lavender, lemon, and peppermint in 2tsp of honey. mmmmm!

or

Apply topically one drop of lavendar, lemon, & peppermint on feet, OR behind ears, back of the neck, and across their nose.

TOP 30 OILS FOR YOUR ALLERGIES

This chapter is going to examine in detail, a list of essential oils that can help you – or your loved ones – with allergies. Of course, there are hundreds and which ones you will like depend on your allergy and your individual situation – this list is simple a guideline of the top 30 to get you started.

1. Clary Sage

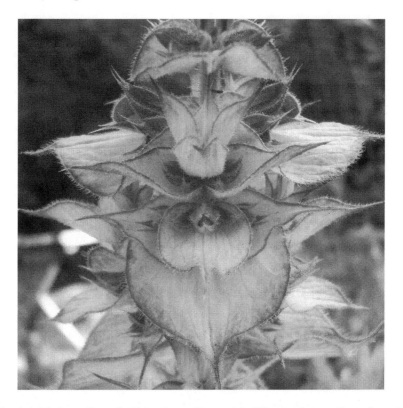

The health benefits of Clary Sage Essential Oil can be attributed to its properties as an antidepressant, anticonvulsive, antispasmodic, antiseptic, aphrodisiac, astringent, bactericidal, carminative, deodorant, digestive, emenagogue, euphoric, hypotensive, nervine, sedative, stomachic and uterine substance.

Clary Sage Essential Oil is extracted by steam distillation from the buds and leaves of the Clary Sage plant whose scientific name is Salvia Sclarea. It is an herb, believed to be a native species of Europe, which has been highly praised as a medicinal plant throughout history, particularly owing to its numerous benefits for vision and eye health. It is a close relative of common garden sage, but it has a slightly different organic makeup. Furthermore, you may be familiar with it as *"Muscatel Oil"*, a common name given to Clary Sage essential oil due to its traditional use of flavoring muscatel wine.

Latin Name: Salvia sclarea.

Color: Light to golden yellow.

Scent: Bright, earthy, herbaceous, with a subtle fruity note.

Location: Northern Mediterranean, North Africa, Central Asia.

Part of the Plant Used: Leaves and flowers.

Distillation Method: The straight steam method.

Allergies Fought: Clary sage oil regulates oil production and reduces inflammation that contributes to dermatitis. It's to be used topically on the affected area.

Where To Buy: Local specialist or online resources, such as Amazon.com, YoungLiving.com, doTerra.com, iHerb.com.

Notes: Suitable for children, but only in very loses doses.

2. Clove

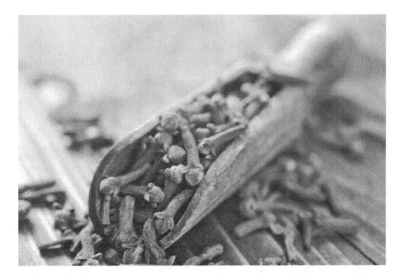

Cloves are the aromatic flower buds of a tree in the family Myrtaceae, Syzygium aromaticum. They are native to the Maluku Islands in Indonesia, and are commonly used as a spice. Cloves are commercially harvested primarily in Indonesia, India, Madagascar, Zanzibar, Pakistan, Sri Lanka and Tanzania.

The clove tree is an evergreen tree that grows up to 8–12 m tall, with large leaves and sanguine flowers grouped in terminal clusters. The flower buds initially have a pale hue, gradually turn green, then transition to a bright red when ready for harvest. Cloves are harvested at 1.5–2.0 cm long, and consist of a long calyx that terminates in four spreading sepals, and four unopened petals that form a small central ball.

Latin Name: Syzygium aromaticum.

Color: Golden yellow to brown.

Scent: Spicy, warm but slightly bitter, woody, richer than clove buds.

Location: Indonesia.

Part of the Plant Used: Buds.

Distillation Method: The straight steam method.

Allergies Fought: Clove oil is anti-inflammatory and anti-microbial, and can help to reduce allergy symptoms for hay fever and asthma. It's most effective when used aromatically – in a diffuser or in the bath.

Where To Buy: Local specialist or online resources, such as Amazon.com, YoungLiving.com, doTerra.com, iHerb.com.

Notes: Avoid use with children under 2. Do not use if allergic to eugenol, suffer from Crohn's disease or have liver problems. Avoid use of cloves and clove oil during pregnancy.

3. Cypress

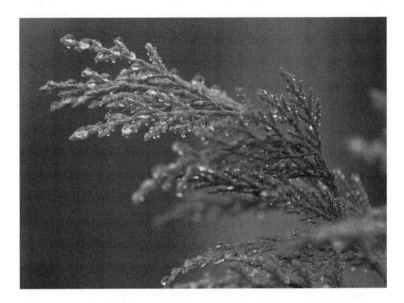

The health benefits of Cypress Essential Oil can be attributed to its properties as an astringent, antiseptic, antispasmodic, deodorant, diuretic, hemostatic, hepatic, styptic, sudorific, vasoconstricting, respiratory tonic and sedative substance.

The Essential Oil of Cypress is obtained through steam distillation of young twigs, stems and needles. Cypress, a needle bearing tree of Coniferous and Deciduous regions, bears the scientific name of *Cupressus Sempervirens*.

The essential oils extracted from Cypress contain components like Alpha Pinene, Beta Pinene, Alpha Terpinene, Bornyl Acetate, Carene, Camphene, Cedrol, Cadinene, Sabinene, Myrcene, Terpinolene and Linalool, which contribute to its medicinal properties. Although the Cypress tree is often linked with death and is commonly found in and around cemeteries, the essential oil obtained from this tree can save you from some truly devastating conditions and illnesses.

Latin Name: Cupressaceae.

Color: Pale yellow.

Scent: Fresh, herbaceous, woody.

Location: South East USA.

Part of the Plant Used: Needles.

Distillation Method: The straight steam method.

Allergies Fought: Antispasmodic and disinfectant. Helps to relieve breathing difficulties and suppress coughing. May benefit symptoms of Asthma. It's is best used aromatically.

Where To Buy: Local specialist or online resources, such as Amazon.com, YoungLiving.com, doTerra.com, iHerb.com, NowFoods.com.

Notes: Do not use on very young children.

4. Elemi

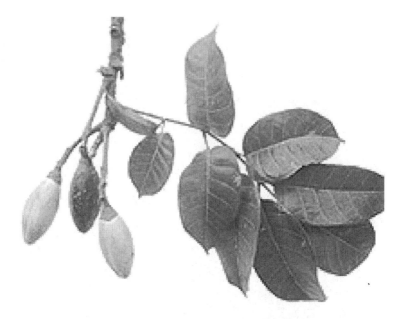

Canarium luzonicum, commonly known as elemi, is a tree native to the Philippines. The oleoresin harvested from it is also known as elemi. Elemi resin is a pale yellow substance, of honey-like consistency. Aromatic elemi oil is steam distilled from the resin. It is a fragrant resin with a sharp pine and lemon-like scent. One of the resin components is called *amyrin*.

Elemi resin is chiefly used commercially in varnishes and lacquers, and certain printing inks. It is used as a herbal medicine to treat bronchitis, catarrh, extreme coughing, mature skin, scars, stress, and wounds.

Latin Name: Canarium luzonicum.

Color: Clear with a tinge of yellow.

Scent: Fresh, citrusy, peppery, spicy.

Location: Philippines.

Part of the Plant Used: Resin.

Distillation Method: The straight steam method.

Allergies Fought: Elemi is anti-infectious, antiseptic and works to calm animal allergies. It is best used in a diffuser.

Where To Buy: Local specialist or online resources, such as Amazon.com, YoungLiving.com, EdensGarden.com, HopeWell.com.

Notes: Suitable for children, but only in very loses doses.

5. Oregano

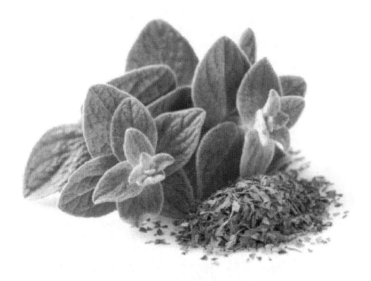

Oregano oil is derived from the leaves and flowers of oregano, a hardy, bushy perennial herb, and a member of the mint (*Lamiaceae*) family. It's native to Europe, although it grows in many areas around the world. The plant grows up to 90 centimeters (35 inches) high, with dark green leaves that are two to three centimeters long.

The ancient Greeks and Romans have a profound appreciation for oregano, using it for various medicinal uses. In fact, its name comes from the Greek words "oros" and "ganos," which are words for mountain and joy, oregano literally means "joy of the mountain." It was revered as a symbol of happiness, and it was an ancient tradition to crown brides and grooms with a laurel of oregano.

Latin Name: Origanum vulgare.

Color: Pale yellow.

Scent: Herbaceous, sharp.

Location: Greece, India.

Part of the Plant Used: Leaves, flowers and buds.

Distillation Method: The straight steam method.

Allergies Fought: Oregano oil can produce sedating effect on the hyper-sensitivity of allergies, which ultimately encourages relief. The most common allergies helped are animals, perfume, cosmetics, dust. It is most effective when used aromatically.

Where To Buy: Local specialist or online resources, such as Amazon.com, iHerb.com, YoungLiving.com, MountainRoseHerbs.com.

Notes: Avoid topical use with children under 5.

6. Frankincense

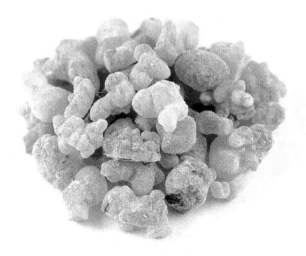

Frankincense, also known as *olibanum*, comes from the *Boswellia* genustrees, particularly *Boswellia sacra* and *Boswellia carteri*. The milky white sap is extracted from the tree bark, allowed to harden into a gum resin for several days, and then scraped off in tear-shaped droplets.

Boswellia trees grow in African and Arabian regions, including Yemen, Oman, Somalia, and Ethiopia. Oman is the best known and most ancient source of frankincense, where it's been traded and shipped to other places like the Mediterranean, India, and China for thousands of years.

Latin Name: Boswellia.

Color: Light yellow.

Scent: Fresh, woody, balsamic, mildly spicy, fruity.

Location: Africa, Arabia.

Part of the Plant Used: Resin.

Distillation Method: The straight steam method.

Allergies Fought: Studies have demonstrated that frankincense has immune enhancing abilities which may help destroy dangerous bacteria, viruses, and skin allergies. It's most effective when used topically on the affected area.

Where To Buy: Local specialist or online resources, such as Amazon.com, iHerb.com, YoungLiving.com, NativeAmericanNutritionals.com.

Notes: Suitable for children, but only in very loses doses.

7. Lemongrass

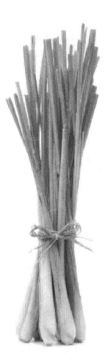

Lemongrass is a plant that is commonly used in Asian cuisine but which may provide therapeutic and medical benefits. Easily available from any ethnic store, health food store, online merchant or in the seasoning aisle of the supermarket, its anti-bacterial, anti-microbial, antioxidant and therapeutic properties make lemongrass a useful alternative or complementary remedy for a wide spectrum of common ailments. Whether using the dried leaves steeped to make tea or the extracted essential oil, lemongrass produces considerable benefits.

The main chemical component found in lemongrass is citral, an aromatic compound, also known as lemonal. Citral is used in perfumes because of its lemon odor. It is the presence of citral which accounts for lemongrass' lemon scent. It is an antimicrobial and therefore effective in destroying or inhibiting microorganisms. Citral also contains antifungal properties. This chemical has pheromonal qualities, which explains its industrial use as an insect repellant. It also has a positive effective on the body's ability to use Vitamin A. The compounds myrcene, citronellal, geranyl acetate, nerol and geraniol are found in varying quantities in Citral. Myrcene, geraniol and nerol contribute to lemongrass' strong fragrance, *citronella* acts as an insecticide and geranyl acetate is another flavoring agent. Lemongrass has rubefacient properties, meaning that it may be able to improve blood circulation.

Latin Name: Cymbopogon.

Color: Pale to vivid yellow.

Scent: Fresh, lemony, earthy.

Location: Asia.

Part of the Plant Used: Grass.

Distillation Method: The straight steam method.

Allergies Fought: Lemongrass Oil is a tonic in a very clear sense. It tones all the systems functioning in the body, such as respiratory system, digestive system, nervous system and excretory system and facilitates absorption of nutrients into the body, thus providing strength and boosting the immune system and fighting food allergies. It can also help to clear oily skin and acne, as well as relieve painful or itchy skin. It works well when used aromatically or topically.

Where To Buy: Local specialist or online resources, such as Amazon.com, iHerb.com, YoungLiving.com, MountainRoseHerbs.com.

Notes: Avoid topical use for children under 2.

8. Spearmint

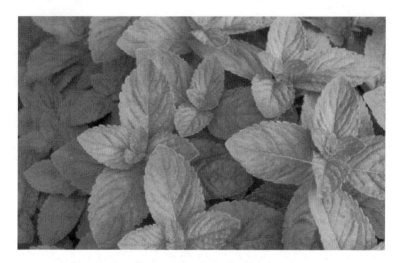

The use of spearmint oil dates back to ancient times. This perennial herb originated from the Mediterranean region. In Ayurvedic medicine, it was used to treat digestive conditions, skin problems, and headaches. The historical record shows that it was used extensively ancient Greece. It was added to baths and used to treat sexually transmitted diseases, whiten teeth, and heal mouth sores.

In modern times, this essential oil is still widely used as a cure for digestive discomfort, as well as for menstrual problems and nausea.

Latin Name: Mentha spicata.

Color: Clear.

Scent: Minty and slightly fruity.

Location: Europe, Asia.

Part of the Plant Used: Leaves, flowers and buds.

Distillation Method: The straight steam method.

Allergies Fought: The therapeutic properties of spearmint oil are antiseptic, antispasmodic, carminative, cephalic, emmenagogue, insecticide, restorative and stimulant. It is very useful to deal with digestive problems including the side effects of food allergies, flatulence, constipation, diarrhea

118

and nausea, as it relaxes the stomach muscles and also relieves hiccups. It's very effective when used aromatically or made into a tea.

Where To Buy: Local specialist or online resources, such as Amazon.com, iHerb.com, YoungLiving.com, NowFoods.com.

Notes: Suitable for children, but only in very loses doses.

9. Eucalyptus

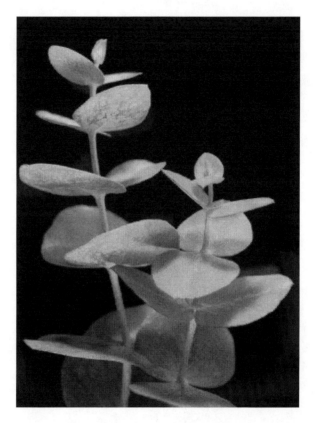

The health benefits of eucalyptus oil are well-known and wide ranging, and its properties include anti-inflammatory, antispasmodic, decongestant, deodorant, antiseptic, antibacterial, stimulating, and other medicinal qualities. Eucalyptus essential oil is colorless and has a distinctive taste and odor.

Though eucalyptus essential oil has most of the properties of a typical volatile oil, it's not very popular as an aromatherapy oil because little was known about it until recent centuries, rather than the more ancient aromatherapy substances. The numerous health benefits of eucalyptus oil have attracted the attention of the entire world, and it has stimulated a great deal of exploration into its usage in aromatherapy as well as in conventional medicine.

Latin Name: Eucalyptus Radiata.

Color: Clear.

Scent: Fresh, medicinal, earthy, woody.

Location: Australia, Indonesia, Philippines.

Part of the Plant Used: Leaves.

Distillation Method: The straight steam method.

Allergies Fought: Eucalyptus helps to fight symptoms such as congestion, headaches and respiratory conditions. It is anti-inflammatory, disinfectant, and expectorant. It can also kill dust mites, a common household allergen. It's most effective when used aromatically.

TIP: You can apply few drops eucalyptus essential oil diluted in a carrier oil onto your neck, chest and bottom of your feet. For inhalation, pour boiling water in a bowl and add few drops of eucalyptus essential oil. Drape the towel over your head and breathe the steam.

Where To Buy: Local specialist or online resources, such as Amazon.com, YoungLiving.com, EdensGarden.com, iHerb.com.

Notes: Avoid use with children under 10.

10. Ginger

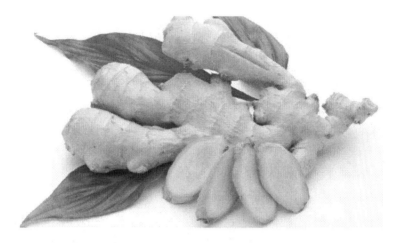

Warm, spicy, and energizing, ginger oil comes from ginger root (*Zingiber officinale*), a pungent, peculiar-looking underground rhizome. A member of the Zingiberaceae plant family, this perennial herb grows up to three to four feet high, with narrow spear-shaped leaves, white or yellow flowers, and small tuberous rhizomes with a thick or thin brown skin. Its flesh can be yellow, white, or red, depending on the variety.

Ginger has been valued for thousands of years for its medicinal and culinary properties, particularly in ancient Chinese, Indian, and Greek civilizations. The *Mahabharata*, a 4th century BC Indian Sanskrit epic, even describes a stewed meat dish that uses ginger as an ingredient. In Ayurvedic medicine, ginger is considered a key plant.

Latin Name: Zingiber officinale.

Color: Light yellow.

Scent: Warm, spicy, earthy, woody.

Location: Asia, West Africa.

Part of the Plant Used: Roots.

Distillation Method: The straight steam method.

Allergies Fought: Analgesic, expectorant and stimulant. Decreases respiratory symptoms such as constricted breathing, wheezing and coughing. Can be very beneficial for any kind of digestive issue or upset stomach, including the side effects of food allergies. It's best used aromatically.

Where To Buy: Local specialist or online resources, such as Amazon.com, iHerb.com, YoungLiving.com, MountainRoseHerbs.com.

Notes: Avoid topical use with children under 2.

11. Lemon

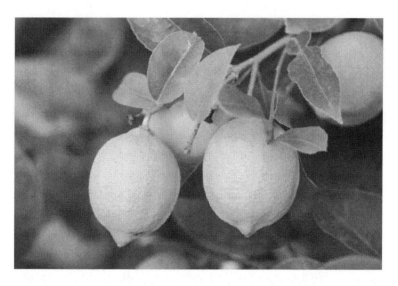

A lemon is a small evergreen tree native to Asia. The tree's ellipsoidal yellow fruit is used for culinary and non-culinary purposes throughout the world, primarily for its juice, though the pulp and rind (zest) are also used in cooking and baking. The juice of the lemon is about 5% to 6% citric acid, giving the fruit its distinctive, sour taste and making it a key ingredient in drinks and foods such as lemonade and lemon meringue pie.

Latin Name: Citrus limon.

Color: Pale to dark yellow.

Scent: Fresh concentrated lemon.

Location: Asia.

Part of the Plant Used: Peel.

Distillation Method: Cold pressed.

Allergies Fought: Lemon protects immunity, relieves respiratory issues such as asthma and hay fever. Excellent antibacterial agent, which makes it well suited for respiratory inflammation. It is most effective when used aromatically, particularly in a diffuser.

TIP: Always dilute lemon oil in a carrier oil before using it for your skin. Do not use it before exposed to sunlight.

Where To Buy: Local specialist or online resources, such as Amazon.com, YoungLiving.com, iHerb.com, HopeWellOils.com.

Notes: Avoid topical use for children under 2.

12. Peppermint

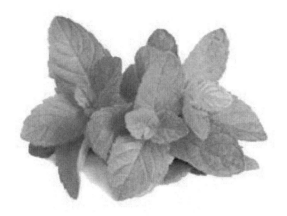

Peppermint is a hybrid mint, a cross between watermint and spearmint. The plant, indigenous to Europe and the Middle East, is now widespread in cultivation in many regions of the world. It is found wild occasionally with its parent species. Peppermint typically occurs in moist habitats, including stream sides and drainage ditches. Being a hybrid, it is usually sterile, producing no seeds and reproducing only vegetatively, spreading by its rhizomes. If placed, it can grow anywhere, with a few exceptions.

Outside of its native range, areas where peppermint was formerly grown for oil often have an abundance of feral plants, and it is considered invasive in Australia, the Galápagos Islands, New Zealand, and in the United States in the Great Lakes region, noted since 1843.

Latin Name: Mentha piperita.

Color: Clear with a yellow tinge.

Scent: Strong, minty.

Location: Europe, Asia.

Part of the Plant Used: Ariel parts.

Distillation Method: The straight steam method.

Allergies Fought: Peppermint helps to improve breathing by opening sinuses and airways, fights infection, relieves pain of headache and muscular pain, and has anti-inflammatory properties so is perfect for asthma and respiratory allergies. It is best used aromatically.

TIP: Add 1 drop of peppermint essential oil to the base of your neck 2 times a day. To relieve sinus congestion, add 1 drop of peppermint essential oil in a carrier oil and apply around your nostrils. To make a chest rub, dilute 2 to 3 drops in a carrier oil of your liking and massage your chest for a few minutes to find relief. To clear sinus congestion, pour boiling water in a bowl and add few drops of peppermint oil. Drape a towel over your head and breathe the steam.

Where To Buy: Local specialist or online resources, such as Amazon.com, YoungLiving.com, iHerb.com, MountainRoseHerbs.com.

Notes: Do not take if you're suffering from gallbladder disease or achlorhydria. Avoid during pregnancy or breast feeding. Avoid use with children under 6.

13. Ravensara

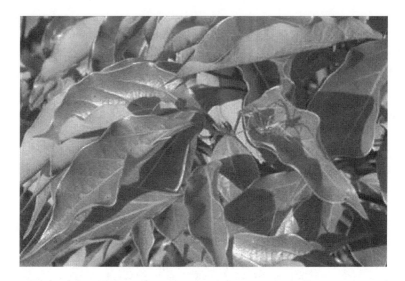

The health benefits of Ravensara Essential Oil can be attributed to its properties as an analgesic, anti-allergenic, antibacterial, antimicrobial, antidepressant, antifungal, antiseptic, antispasmodic, antiviral, aphrodisiac, disinfectant, diuretic, expectorant, relaxant and tonic substance.

Ravensara essential oil is a powerful oil from the mysterious island of Madagascar, that beautiful spot off the Eastern coast of Africa. Ravensara is a large rainforest tree native to Madagascar and its botanical name is *Ravensara Aromatica*. Its essential oil is praised in Madagascar as a "Cure All" oil, in much the same way as tea tree oil is heralded in Australia.

Latin Name: Ravensara Aromatica.

Color: Clear with a tinge of yellow.

Scent: Slightly medicinal, sweet with a fruity hint.

Location: Madagascar.

Part of the Plant Used: Leaves.

Distillation Method: The straight steam method.

Allergies Fought: Ravensara oil has anti-allergenic properties as it is non-sensitizing and non-irritating. It is effective in preventing as well as reducing allergies. It helps your body build a gradual resistance to allergenic substances and thus reduce your predisposition to allergy. It's mostly used for dermatitis and other skin allergies. It is most effective when used topically on the affected area.

Where To Buy: Local specialist or online resources, such as Amazon.com, doTerra.com, MountainRoseHerbs.com.

Notes: Suitable for children, but only in very loses doses.

14. Roman Chamomile

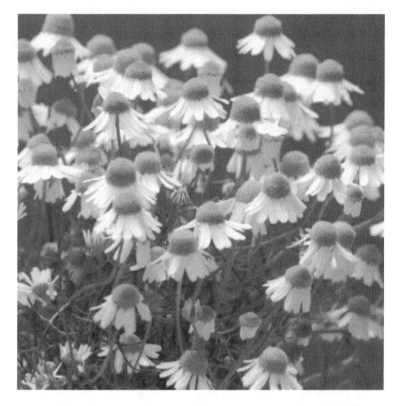

Roman Chamomile has daisy-like white flowers and procumbent stems; the leaves are alternate, bipinnate, finely dissected, and downy to glabrous. The solitary, terminal flowerheads, rising 20–30 cm (8–12 in) above the ground, consist of prominent yellow disk flowers and silver-white ray flowers. The flowering time is June and July, and its fragrance is sweet, crisp, fruity and herbaceous.

Latin Name: Chamaemelum nobile.

Color: Grey or very pale blue.

Scent: Bright, crisp, sweet, fruity, herbaceous.

Location: Northwestern Europe, North Ireland.

Part of the Plant Used: Flowers.

Distillation Method: The straight steam method.

Allergies Fought: Roman chamomile contains chemicals that can help decrease gas (flatulence), relax muscles, and cause sedation which makes it perfect for the side effects of food allergies. It's best used to fight allergies aromatically. It also works wonders to treat rashes, eczema and other skin conditions caused by allergic reaction.

TIP: Dilute a few drops in a carrier oil such as jojoba, coconut or olive oil. Apply on the affected areas three times a day.

Where To Buy: Local specialist or online resources, such as Amazon.com, YoungLiving.com, NativeAmericanNutritionals.com, HopeWellOils.com.

Notes: Suitable for children, but only in very loses doses.

15. Rosemary

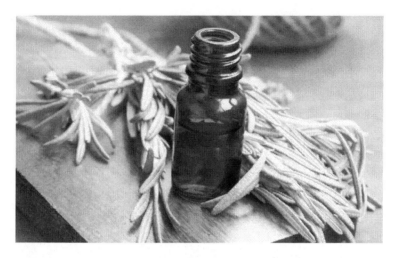

Related to mint and looking like lavender, rosemary has leaves like flat pine needles touched with silver. It boasts of a woodsy, citrus-like fragrance that has become a feature of many kitchens, gardens, and apothecaries worldwide. It derives its name from Latin words *ros* ("dew") and *marinus* ("sea"), or "dew of the sea."

The Virgin Mary is said to have spread her blue cloak over a rosemary bush as she rested, and the white flowers turned blue. The shrub came to be known as the "Rose of Mary." Rosemary was considered sacred by the Egyptians, Hebrews, Greeks, and Romans, and was used in the Middle Ages to ward off evil spirits and protect against the plague.

Latin Name: Rosmarinus officinalis.

Color: Clear.

Scent: Fresh, herbaceous, sweet, slightly medicinal.

Location: Mediterranean.

Part of the Plant Used: Leaves, flowers and buds.

Distillation Method: The straight steam method.

Allergies Fought: The scent of Rosemary oil has been shown to give relief from throat congestion, and it is also used in the treatment of respiratory allergies, colds, sore throats, and the flu. It's best used aromatically.

Where To Buy: Local specialist or online resources, such as Amazon.com, iHerb.com, YoungLiving.com, NowFoods.com.

Notes: Avoid use with children under 6. Do not take if you have an allergy to aspirin, suffer from bleeding disorders, epilepsy, high blood pressure, ulcers, colitis or if you're pregnant, breast feeding or trying to conceive.

16. Tea Tree

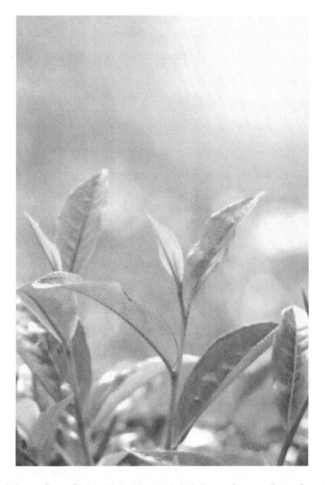

The health benefits of Tea Tree Essential Oil can be attributed to its properties as an antibacterial, antimicrobial, antiseptic, antiviral, balsamic, cicatrisant, expectorant, fungicide, insecticide, stimulant and sudorific substance.

Unlike the name suggests, the essential oil of Tea Tree is not extracted from the plant commonly associated with tea as a beverage. Neither is it related to Tea Oil, which is extracted from the seed of the Tea plant. Instead, it is extracted through steam distillation of twigs and leaves of Tea Tree, which has the botanical name Melaleuca Alternifolia. The tea tree is native to Southeast Queensland and New South Wales, in Australia, which is why it is such a common and popular essential oil in that country. However, its impressive qualities have spread to other parts of the world, so it cannot be found internationally.

Latin Name: Melaleuca Alternifolia.

Color: Clear with a yellow tinge.

Scent: Medicinal, earthy, woody, herbaceous, fresh.

Location: Australia.

Part of the Plant Used: Leaves.

Distillation Method: The straight steam method.

Allergies Fought: There are over 100 components in tea tree oil, but it is mostly made up of terpene hydrocarbons: monoterpenes, sesquiterpenes, and their alcohol which work towards soothing skin allergies, such as eczema, dermatitis or psoriasis. Tea tree oil is best used topically on the affected area.

Where To Buy: Local specialist or online resources, such as Amazon.com, iHerb.com, YoungLiving.com, EdensGarden.com.

Notes: Avoid topical use with children under 2.

17. Lavender

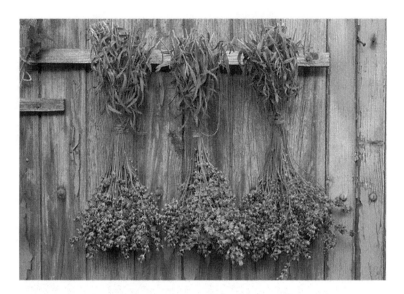

Lavender is an evergreen and fragrant shrub native to southern Europe, especially around the Mediterranean. The majority of the commercial crop is grown in France, Spain, Bulgaria and the Soviet Union. Some is also grown in Tasmania, and there is a minor, but flourishing, industry in Norfolk, England.

Lavender can grow at considerable heights – one organic Provencal grower calls his product 'Lavande 1100' from the height in metres (3,600 ft) at which his plants are cultivated. Individual lavender plants grow up to 1 m (3 ft) in height, and can become very woody and spreading. The narrow leaves are grey and downy; the flowers are blue-grey, borne on long slender stems. The oil glands are in tiny star-shaped hairs with which the leaves, flowers and stems are covered; rub a flower or leaf between your fingers to release some oil (it has a short-lived aroma).

Latin Name: Lavandula angustifolia.

Color: Clear with a tinge of yellow.

Scent: Floral, fresh, sweet, herbaceous and sometimes fruity.

Location: Primarily Tasmania.

Part of the Plant Used: Flowers, buds and leaves.

Distillation Method: The straight steam method.

Allergies Fought: Lavender EO works as a natural antihistamine and possess strong anti-inflammatory properties to treat and relief most allergic reactions, including insect bites. Works great to treat skin rashes or headaches. And not only will it ease your allergic reaction, it has a calming and relaxing effect on body and mind and is best taken aromatically.

TIP: Add 1 drop of lavender to your cheeks, forehead, and sinuses as needed to soothe allergic reactions or headaches. Before bed, add a few drops to the soles of your feet. For skin rashes or itchy skin, dilute a few drops of lavender essential oil in a carrier oil and rub onto the affected areas 3 times a day. Alternatively you can use lavender essential oil in cold diffuser. Diffuse for 15 minutes every two hours for the best effect or next to your bed during night time.

Where To Buy: Local specialist or online resources, such as Amazon.com, YoungLiving.com, doTerra.com.

Notes: Suitable for children, but only in very loses doses.

18. Coriander

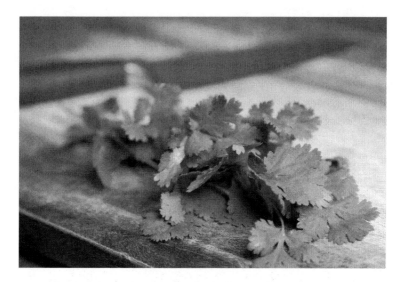

The health benefits of Coriander Essential Oil can be attributed to its properties as an analgesic, aphrodisiac, antispasmodic, carminative, depurative, deodorant, digestive, fungicidal, lipolytic, stimulant and stomachic substance.

Coriander essential oil is extracted from the seeds of coriander with the help of steam distillation. The scientific name of Coriander is Coriandrum Sativum. Coriander essential oil consists of compounds like Borneol, Cineole, Cymene, Dipentene, Linalool, Phellandrene, Pinene, Terpineol and Terpinolene, and these are the causes behind its medicinal properties.

Latin Name: Coriandrum sativum.

Color: Pale yellow.

Scent: Sweet, herbaceous, woody, spicy, slightly fruity.

Location: Southern Europe, Northern Africa, Southwestern Asia.

Part of the Plant Used: Seeds.

Distillation Method: The straight steam method.

Allergies Fought: Antispasmodic and disinfectant. Helps to relieve breathing difficulties and suppress coughing. Can also help to soothe skin allergies. May benefit symptoms of Asthma when used aromatically.

Where To Buy: Local specialist or online resources, such as Amazon.com, iHerb.com, YoungLiving.com, MountainRoseHerbs.com.

Notes: Avoid use with very young children.

19. Cajeput

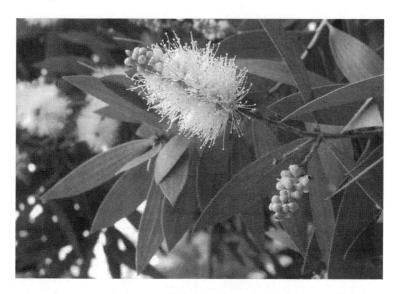

Cajeput oil is a volatile oil obtained by distillation from the leaves of the myrtaceous trees Melaleuca leucadendra, Melaleuca cajuputi, and probably other Melaleuca species. The trees yielding the oil are found throughout Maritime Southeast Asia and over the hotter parts of the Australian continent. The majority of the oil is produced on the Indonesian island of Sulawesi. The name "cajeput" is derived from its Indonesian name, "kayu putih" or "white wood".

The oil is prepared from leaves collected on a hot dry day, macerated in water, and distilled after fermenting for a night. This oil is extremely pungent, and has the odor of a mixture of turpentine and camphor. It consists mainly of cineol (see terpenes), from which cajuputene, having a hyacinth-like odor, can be obtained by distillation with phosphorus pentoxide. The drug is a typical volatile oil, and is used internally in doses of 2 to 3 minims, for the same purposes as, say, clove oil. It is frequently employed externally as a counterirritant. It is an ingredient in some liniments for sore muscles such as Tiger Balm and Indonesian traditional medicine Minyak Telon.

Latin Name: Melaleuca leucadendron.

Color: Clear with a yellow tinge.

Scent: Fresh, campherous aroma with a fruity note.

Location: Indonesia.

Part of the Plant Used: Leaves.

Distillation Method: The straight steam method.

Allergies Fought: Cajeput oil contains a chemical called cineole. When applied to the skin, cineole can cause surface warmth and irritation, which relieves pain beneath the skin, so it works well for skin allergies. It's best used topically on the affected area.

Where To Buy: Local specialist or online resources, such as Amazon.com, EdensGarden.com, MountainRoseHerbs.com, doTerra.com.

Notes: Avoid use with children under 6.

20. Grapefruit

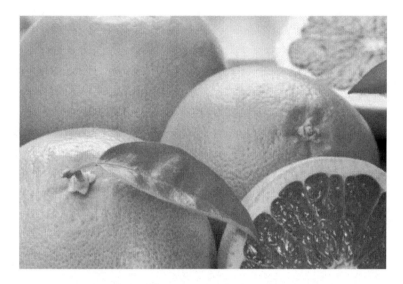

Grapefruit is an excellent source of vitamin C, a vitamin that helps to support the immune system. Vitamin C-rich foods like grapefruit may help reduce cold symptoms or severity of cold symptoms; over 20 scientific studies have suggested that vitamin C is a cold-fighter. Vitamin C also prevents the free radical damage that triggers the inflammatory cascade, and is therefore also associated with reduced severity of inflammatory conditions, such as asthma, osteoarthritis, and rheumatoid arthritis. As free radicals can oxidize cholesterol and lead to plaques that may rupture causing heart attacks or stroke, vitamin C is beneficial to promoting cardiovascular health. Owing to the multitude of vitamin C's health benefits, it is not surprising that research has shown that consumption of vegetables and fruits high in this nutrient is associated with a reduced risk of death from all causes including heart disease, stroke and cancer.

Latin Name: Citrus Paradisi.

Color: Pale yellow to yellow.

Scent: Citrusy, sweeter more concentrated smell of grapefruit.

Location: Barbados.

Part of the Plant Used: Peel.

Distillation Method: Cold pressed.

Allergies Fought: The major components of the essential oil of grapefruit are linalool, thujene, myrcene, terpinene, pinene, citronellol, caprinaldehyde, decyl acetate, and neryl acetate which means it works well for food allergies - specifically wheat. It's most effective for allergies when used aromatically.

Where To Buy: Local specialist or online resources, such as Amazon.com, iHerb.com, YoungLiving.com, doTerra.com.

Notes: Suitable for children, but only in very loses doses.

21. Cinnamon

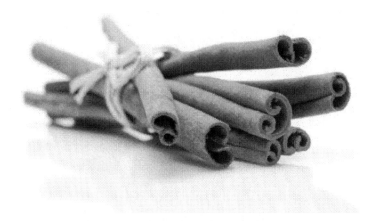

Cinnamon is a spice obtained from the inner bark of several trees from the genus Cinnamomum that is used in both sweet and savory foods. While Cinnamomum verum is sometimes considered to be "true cinnamon", most cinnamon in international commerce is derived from related species, which are also referred to as "cassia" to distinguish them from "true cinnamon".

Cinnamon is the name for perhaps a dozen species of trees and the commercial spice products that some of them produce. All are members of the genus Cinnamomum in the family Lauraceae. Only a few of them are grown commercially for spice.

Latin Name: Cinnamomum zeylanicum.

Color: Golden yellow to brown.

Scent: Richer aroma than ground cinnamon.

Location: Asia.

Part of the Plant Used: Leaf or bark.

Distillation Method: The straight steam method.

Allergies Fought: Cinnamon oil owes its medicinal properties to its alcohol and aldehyde content, which makes it perfect for fighting the side effects of food allergies. It's best used aromatically.

Where To Buy: Local specialist or online resources, such as Amazon.com, iHerb.com, YoungLiving.com, doTerra.com.

Notes: Suitable for children, but only in very loses doses.

22. Myrrh

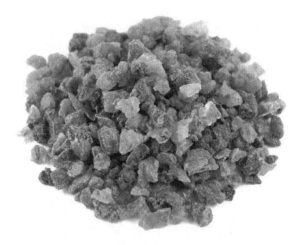

Myrrh is the aromatic resin of a number of small, thorny tree species of the genus Commiphora, which is an essential oil termed an oleoresin. Myrrh resin is a natural gum. It has been used throughout history as a perfume, incense and medicine. It can also be ingested by mixing it with wine.

When a tree wound penetrates through the bark and into the sapwood, the tree bleeds a resin. Myrrh gum, like frankincense, is such a resin. When people harvest myrrh, they wound the trees repeatedly to bleed them of the gum. Myrrh gum is waxy, and coagulates quickly. After the harvest, the gum becomes hard and glossy. The gum is yellowish, and may be either clear or opaque. It darkens deeply as it ages, and white streaks emerge.

Latin Name: Commiphora Molmol.

Color: Golden yellow or brown.

Scent: Warm, earthy, woody, balsamic.

Location: Yemen.

Part of the Plant Used: Resin.

Distillation Method: The straight steam method.

Allergies Fought: There are many health-enhancing compounds in myrrh oil, such as terpenoids, a class of chemicals with anti-inflammatory and antioxidant effects. If impacts on your hormones and works well in the fight against animal allergies. It's most effective when used aromatically.

Where To Buy: Local specialist or online resources, such as Amazon.com, YoungLiving.com, MountainRoseHerbs.com, EdensGarden.com.

Notes: Suitable for children, but only in very loses doses.

23. Sandalwood

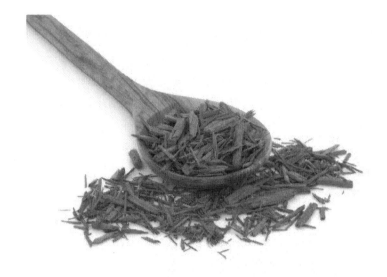

The health benefits of Sandalwood essential oil can be attributed to its properties as an antiseptic, anti-inflammatory, antiphlogistic, antispasmodic, astringent, cicatrisant, carminative, diuretic, disinfectant, emollient, expectorant, hypotensive, memory booster, sedative and tonic substance.

The essential oil of sandalwood is extracted through steam distillation of pieces of wood from matured Sandalwood trees which are 40-80 years old, although 80 years is preferred. The older the tree, the more oil is available, and the aroma is stronger.

Latin Name: Santalum album.

Color: Clear to pale yellow.

Scent: Rich, sweet, fragrant, woody, floral.

Location: Europe, India, Asia.

Part of the Plant Used: Wood.

Distillation Method: The straight steam method.

Allergies Fought: This essential oil is well-regarded in skincare, as it tones and relieves itching, inflammation, and dehydrated skin. Rashes, scar tissue, eczema, psoriasis, acne, allergies and dandruff are just some of the issues it can assist with. It is most effective when applied topically to the affected area.

Where To Buy: Local specialist or online resources, such as Amazon.com, iHerb.com, YoungLiving.com, MountainRoseHerbs.com.

Notes: Suitable for children, but only in very loses doses.

24. Geranium

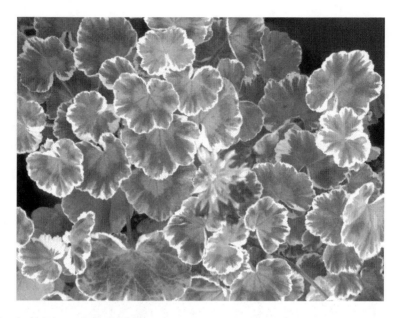

The health benefits of Geranium Essential Oil can be attributed to its properties as an astringent, hemostatic, cicatrisant, cytophylactic, diuretic, deodorant, styptic, tonic, vermifuge and vulnerary agent. It is widely used as an element in aromatherapy for its many health benefits, including its ability to balance hormones, relieve stress and depression, reduce inflammation and irritation, improve the health of the skin, alleviate the effects of menopause, improve circulation, benefit dental health, boost kidney health, and reduce blood pressure.

Latin Name: Pelargonium.

Color: Ranges from clear to amber.

Scent: Floral, fresh, sweet, slightly fruity.

Location: Eastern Mediterranean.

Part of the Plant Used: Leaves.

Distillation Method: The straight steam method.

Allergies Fought: Geranium oil also functions to reduce pain and inflammation. Its antiseptic properties can help speed up the healing of wounds and treat a variety of skin problems, such as burns, frostbite, fungal infections, athlete's foot, and eczema. It's very effective when applied topically to the affected area.

Where To Buy: Local specialist or online resources, such as Amazon.com, iHerb.com, YoungLiving.com, HopeWellOils.com.

Notes: Suitable for children, but only in very loses doses.

25. Cedarwood

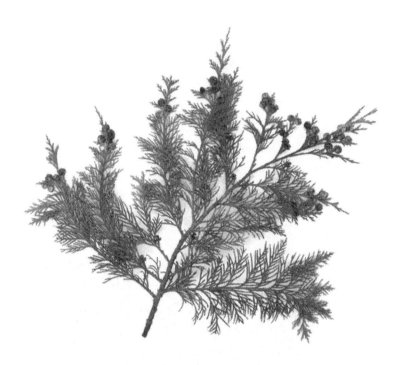

Cedar oil, also known as cedarwood oil, is an essential oil derived from the foliage, and sometimes the wood and roots, of various types of conifers, most in the pine or cypress botanical families. It has many uses in medicine, art, industry and perfumery, and while the characteristics of oils derived from various species may themselves vary, all have some degree of bactericidal and pesticidal effects.

Although termed cedar or cedarwood oils, the most important oils of this group are produced from distilling wood of a number of different junipers and cypresses (Juniperus and Cupressus spp., of the family Cupressaceae), rather than true cedars (Cedrus spp., of the family Pinaceae). A cedar leaf oil is also commercially distilled from the Eastern arborvitae (Thuja occidentalis, also of the Cupressaceae), and similar oils are distilled, pressed or chemically extracted in small quantities from wood, roots and leaves from plants of the genera Platycladus, Cupressus, Taiwania and Calocedrus.

Latin Name: Cedrus atlantica.

Color: Light to golden yellow.

Scent: Woody, sweet.

Location: North America.

Part of the Plant Used: Wood.

Distillation Method: The straight steam method.

Allergies Fought: This wonderful essential oil has many, many healing properties, but it is most often used for its tranquilizing effect. Cedar wood oil is also a valuable tool in skin issues such as dermatitis and eczema. It's best used topically, on the affected area.

Where To Buy: Local specialist or online resources, such as Amazon.com, YoungLiving.com, doTerra.com, iHerb.com.

Notes: Suitable for children, but only in very loses doses.

26. Garlic

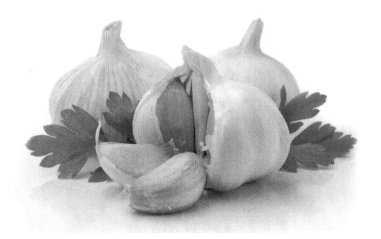

Garlic, especially in its raw form, has been praised for its healing power and medicinal uses since ancient times. It was used for medicinal purposes by the ancient Greeks, Egyptians, Babylonians, Assyrians, Romans and Chinese. Today, numerous research studies document the extraordinary benefits of garlic on human health.

The healing properties of garlic are wide and varied, ranging from antioxidant, antifungal, antiviral and antibacterial properties to cancer-fighting and immune-boosting activity. Due to its healing properties, raw garlic has been used as a medicinal plant to prevent – and in some cases treat or even heal – various health complaints.

Latin Name: Allium sativum.

Color: Clear to pale yellow.

Scent: Potent garlicy smell.

Location: Mexico.

Part of the Plant Used: Bulbs.

Distillation Method: The straight steam method.

Allergies Fought: Garlic is a natural antibiotic that wards off infections, viruses and even allergens, such as dust mites. It's most effective when used aromatically.

Where To Buy: Local specialist or online resources, such as Amazon.com, doTerra.com.

Notes: Avoid topical use with children under 2. Do not take if allergic to garlic. Do not take high doses during pregnancy or breastfeeding. Avoid taking it with anticoagulants or diabetes medication and if you're planning a surgery within next 7 days.

27. Immortelle (Helichrysum)

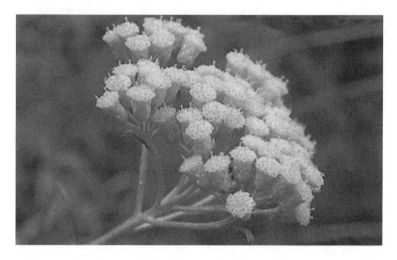

Produced in the Mediterranean countries, Madagascar and France this warm, earthy, rich oil is distilled from the flowers. Known for its anti-inflammatory, analgesic and regenerative properties, this remarkable oil is used in many healing formulas from infection and inflammation in respiratory conditions, muscle pain, arthritis to liver problems and as a detoxifier in drug withdrawal.

Latin Name: Xerochrysum bracteatum.

Color: Light yellow.

Scent: Fresh, earthy, herbaceous.

Location: Mediterranean.

Part of the Plant Used: Flowers.

Distillation Method: The straight steam method.

Allergies Fought: Immortelle is useful skin care oil it being anti-allergenic, anti-inflammatory, and astringent. It promotes new cell growth and has good antioxidant qualities. If you suffer from eczema or any skin irritation, this is perfect when applied topically to the affected area.

Where To Buy: Local specialist or online resources, such as NativeAmericanNutritions.com, MountainRoseHerbs.com, EdensGarden.com.

Notes: Do not use with children under 12 years old.

28. Fennel

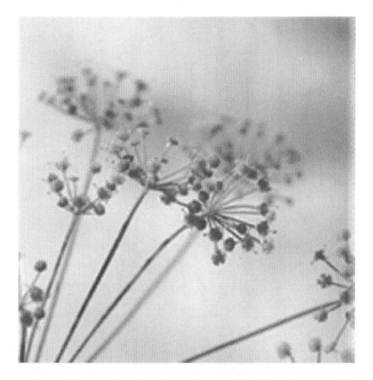

The benefits of fennel date back to the ancient Egyptians and Romans. They used fennel for spiritual and emotional support as well as medicinal reasons. Traditionally they used it for snake bites, lung and kidney support and to balance the female reproductive system. Spiritually warriors believed that it gave them courage and strength in battle and longevity. During the Medieval Age, fennel was used to block spells and ward off witches and evil spirits.

Today, we can reap the benefits of fennel using fennel essential oil every day. It can assist us with any kinds of occasional digestive upset. It also is supportive of the circulatory glandular and respiratory systems.

Latin Name: Foeniculum vulgare.

Color: Clear with a faint yellow tinge.

Scent: Sweet, spicy, like licorice.

Location: Mediterranean.

Part of the Plant Used: Seeds.

Distillation Method: The straight steam method.

Allergies Fought: Fennel relaxes the colon and decrease respiratory tract secretions, helping with the side effects of food allergies. It's great when used aromatically.

Where To Buy: Local specialist or online resources, such as Amazon.com, YoungLiving.com, MountainRoseHerbs.com.

Notes: Avoid use with children under 5.

29. Arborvitae

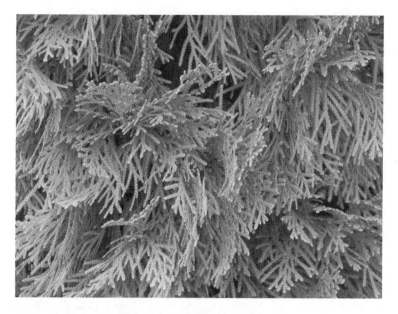

Known as the *"tree of life,"* Arborvitae is majestic in size and abundant in therapeutic benefits. These trees can be thousands of years old, be dead and lying on the ground but still not be deteriorated at all. Arborvitae essential oil has a high content of tropolones, a group of chemical compounds that protect against environmental and seasonal threats, have powerful purifying properties, and promote healthy cell function.

Hinokitiol, one of the tropolones in Arborvitae, protects the body from harmful elements while supporting normal cell activity. This compound also contributes to Arborvitae's natural insect repellent properties. Thujic acid, another tropolone found in Arborvitae, has been studied for its ability to protect against common threats in the environment. Native to Canada, all parts of the Arborvitae tree were used extensively by Native Americans for health benefits and for building vessels, totem poles, baskets, and clothing. Because of its natural preserving properties, Arborvitae prevents wood from rotting, which makes it popular in woodcraft and for preserving natural wood surfaces.

Latin Name: Thuja.

Color: Clear to pale yellow/green.

Scent: Pungent, woody, warm.

Location: Canada.

Part of the Plant Used: Needles and twigs.

Distillation Method: The straight steam method.

Allergies Fought: Antibacterial, antifungal, antiseptic which works well in the side effects of food allergies. It's best used aromatically.

Where To Buy: Local specialist or online resources, such as Amazon.com, EdensGarden.com.

Notes: Suitable for children, but only in very loses doses.

30. Thyme

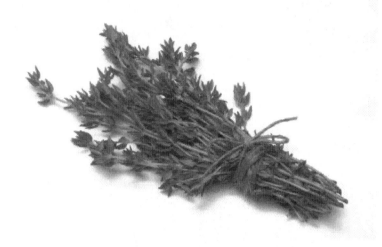

Oil of thyme is derived from thyme, also known as *Thymus vulgaris*. The perennial herb, a member of the mint family, is used in aromatherapy, cooking, potpourri, mouthwashes, and elixirs, as well as added to ointments. Thyme also has a number of medicinal properties, which is due to the herb's essential oils.

The benefits of thyme essential oil have been recognized for thousands of years in Mediterranean countries. This substance is also a common agent in Ayurverdic practice. Today, among the many producers of thyme oil, France, Morocco, and Spain emerge as the primary ones.

Latin Name: Thymus vulgaris.

Color: Reddish brown.

Scent: Fresh, medicinal, herbaceous.

Location: Europe, Morocco.

Part of the Plant Used: Leaves, flowers and buds.

Distillation Method: The straight steam method.

Allergies Fought: Thyme contains chemicals that might help bacterial and fungal infections, and minor irritations. It also relieves smooth muscle spasms, such as coughing and the other side effects of asthma. It works most effectively when used aromatically.

Where To Buy: Local specialist or online resources, such as Amazon.com, iHerb.com, YoungLiving.com, EdensGarden.com.

Notes: Suitable for children, but only in very loses doses.

So now you have a list of essential oils to get you started in your allergy treatment. This list is, of course, not exhaustive, it's just the beginning of what can be used to help you.

Remember that everyone is individual, and your treatment should be treated as such. Just as a variety of traditional medication will be tried to see what suits you, you will need to experiment with essential oils. For safety, don't take the oils internally – at the very least, not until you are very experienced – and always seek medical advice from a health professional before trying any of the recommended oils.

164

ESSENTIAL OILS TO AVOID

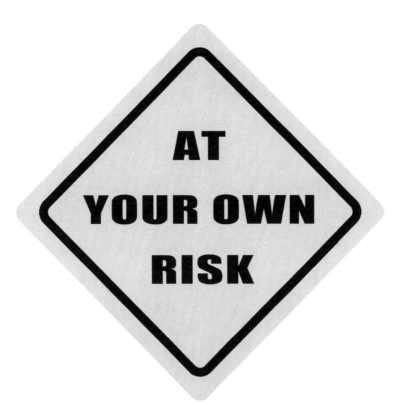

It is widely considered that **essential oils cannot cause or trigger your allergies**, as shown by this statement from Ever Faith:

"Because of the nature of distillation by heat, steam, and water, that true essential oils must undergo, they do not contain the necessary compounds to trigger allergies because these compounds do not pass through the distillation process. Hence, sensitivities to essential oils, in the sense of allergic reactions, are not possible. Allergic sensitivities are due to

the body developing antibodies in response to certain nitrogenous molecules. No one has ever found antibodies in humans from essential oils. So if one has a reaction to an essential oil, it is something else. Not an allergy."

However, whatever your condition – including allergies – it is always advisable to do a **skin patch test** of the essential oils you're thinking about using. Everyone is different and will react to oils in a unique way. You will need to discover what is right for you.

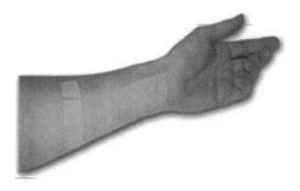

Here is **a patch test guide**:

1. Mix a very small amount of essential oil/carrier at twice the concentration you plan to use. For example, if you plan to use a 3% mixture of the essential oil, mix it at 6% (six drops in a teaspoon of carrier oil, or three drops in 1/2 teaspoon of carrier oil).

2. Using the inside of the forearm, apply a couple drops of your double concentration mix to the pad of a bandaid and keep the bandage on the skin. After 48 hours remove the bandage and check for irritation.

3. You may repeat to check for allergic sensitivity. Remember, however, that allergies can develop any time after the first exposure; thus absence of a reaction does not necessarily mean that an allergy will not develop with later exposures.

4. If the skin under or around the bandage becomes red, swollen, itchy, or develops blisters, that is a reaction and you should avoid skin exposure to the essential oil you tested.

You need to ensure that you **follow all of the instructions on how to use oils,** and Safety Tips to ensure that you get the best from this treatment. It is also very advisable to read all of the ingredients in a product – for example, some products contain almonds, which would be terrible for a nut allergy sufferer. It is *always* best to seek advice from a medical professional before using essential oils.

That being said, there are some **essential oils that are considered unsafe for young children.** Here is a quick guide:

- **Anise/Aniseed** (Pimpinella anisum, Illicium verum) - avoid using (all routes) on children under 5

- **Basil (lemon)** (Ocimum x citriodorum) - avoid topical use on children under 2

- **Benzoin** (Styrax benzoin, Styrax paralleloneurus and Styrax tonkinensis) - avoid topical use on children under 2

- **Birch (sweet)** (Betula lenta) - avoid using (all routes) on children

- **Black Seed** (Nigella sativa) - avoid topical use on children under 2

- **Cajuput** (Melaleuca cajuputi, Melaleuca leucadendron) - avoid using on children under 6

- **Cardamon** (Elettaria cardamomum) - avoid using (all routes) on children under 6

- **Cassia** (Cinnamomum cassia, Cinnamomum aromaticum) - avoid topical use on children under 2

- **Chaste Tree** (Vitex agnus castus) - avoid using (all routes) on prepubertal children

- **Clove Bud, Clove Leaf, Clove Stem** (Syzygium aromaticum, Eugenia caryophyllata, Eugenia aromatica) - avoid topical use on children under 2

- **Cornmint** (Mentha arvensis, Mentha canadensis) - avoid using (all routes) on children under 6

- **Eucalyptus** (Eucalyptus camaldulensis, Eucalyptus globulus, Eucalyptus maidenii, Eucalyptus plenissima, Eucalyptus kochii, Eucalyptus polybractea, Eucalyptus radiata, Eucalyptus Autraliana, Eucalyptus phellandra, Eucalyptus smithii) - avoid using (all routes) on children under 10

- **Fennel (bitter), Fennel (sweet)** (Foeniculum vulgare) - avoid using (all routes) on children under 5

- **Galangal (lesser)** (Alpinia officinarum, Languas officinarum) - avoid using (all routes) on children under 6

- **Garlic** (Allium sativum) - avoid topical use on children under 2

- **Ginger Lily** (Hedychium coronarium) - avoid topical use on children under 2

- **Ho Leaf/Ravintsara** (Cinnamomum camphora) - avoid using on children under 6

- **Hyssop** (Hyssopus officinalis) - avoid using (all routes) on children under 2

- **Laurel Leaf/Bay Laurel** (Laurus nobilis) - avoid topical use on children under 2; avoid all routes for children under age 6

- **Lemon Leaf** (Citrus x limon, Citrus limonum) - avoid topical use on children under 2

- **Lemongrass** (Cymbopogon flexuosus, Andropogon flexuosus, Cymbopogon citratus, Andropogon citratus) - avoid topical use on children under 2

- **Marjoram** (Thymus mastichina) - avoid using (all routes) on children under 6

- **Massoia** (Cryptocarya massoy, Cryptocaria massoia, Massoia aromatica) - avoid using (all routes) on children under 2

- **May Chang** (Litsea cubeba, Litsea citrata, Laura cubeba) - avoid topical use on children under 2

- **Melissa/Lemon Balm** (Melissa officinalis) - avoid topical use on children under 2

- **Myrtle (red)** (Myrtus communis) - avoid using (all routes) on children under 6

- **Myrtle (aniseed)** (Backhousia anisata) - avoid using (all routes) on children under 5

- **Myrtle (honey)** (Melaleuca teretifolia) - avoid topical use on children under 2

- **Myrtle (lemon)/Sweet Verbena** (Backhousia citriodora) - avoid topical use on children under 2

- **Niaouli** (Melaleuca quinquinervia) - avoid using (all routes) on children under 6

- **Oakmoss** (Evernia prunastri) - avoid topical use on children under 2

- **Opopanax** (Commiphora guidottii) - avoid topical use on children under 2

- **Oregano** (Origanum onites, Origanum smyrnaeum, Origanum vulgare, Origanum compactum, Origanum hirtum, Thymbra capitata, Thymus capitatus, Coridothymus capitatus, Satureeja capitata) - avoid topical use on children under 2

- **Peppermint** (Mentha x Piperita) - avoid using (all routes) on children under 6

- **Peru Balsam** (Myroxylon balsamum, Myroxylon pereiraw, Myroxylon peruiferum, Myrospermum pereirae, Toluifera pereirae) - avoid topical use on children under 2

- **Rambiazana** (Helichrysum gymnocephalum) - avoid using (all routes) on children under 6

- **Rosemary** (Rosmarinus officinalis) - avoid using (all routes) on children under 6

- **Saffron** (Crocus sativus) - avoid topical use on children under 2

- **Sage (Greek)** (Salvia fruiticosa, Salvia triloba) - avoid using (all routes) on children under 6

- **Sage (White)** (Salvia apiana) - avoid using (all routes) on children under 6

- **Sage (Wild Mountain)** (Hemizygia petiolata) - avoid topical use on children under 2

- **Sanna** (Hedychium spicatum) - avoid using (all routes) on children under 6

- **Saro** (Cinnamosma fragrans) - avoid using (all routes) on children under 6

- **Savory** (Satureia hortensis, Satureia Montana) - avoid topical use on children under 2

- **Styrax** (Liquidambar orientalis, Liquidambar styraciflua) - avoid topical use on children under 2

- **Tea Leaf/Black Tea** (Camellia sinensis, Thea sinensis) - avoid topical use on children under 2

- **Tea Tree (lemon scented)** (Leptospermum petersonii, Leptospermum citratum, Leptospermum liversidgei) - avoid topical use on children under 2

- **Treemoss** (Pseudevernia furfuracea) - avoid topical use on children under 2

- **Tuberose** (Polianthes tuberose) - avoid topical use on children under 2

- **Turpentine** (Pinus ayacahuite, Pinus caribaea, Pinus contorta, Pinus elliottii, Pinus halepensis, Pinus insularis, Pinus kesiya, Pinus merkusii, Pinus palustris, Pinus pinaster, Pinus radiata, Pinus roxburghii, Pinus tabulaeformis, Pinus teocote, Pinus yunnanensis) - avoid topical use on children under 2

- **Verbena (Lemon)** (Aloysia triphylla, Aloysia citriodora, Lippa citriodora, Lippa triphylla) - avoid topical use on children under 2

- **Wintergreen** (Gaultheria fragrantissima, Gaultheria procumbens) – avoid (all routes) on children due to methyl salicylate content

- **Ylang-Ylang** (Cananga odorata) - avoid topical use on children under 2.

There are also some scenarios in which you should **avoid certain essential oils as an adult**. A lot of these are covered in the <u>Safety</u> chapter of this book.

For extra information on this topic, there are many online resources such as:

Wellness Mama at:

wellnessmama.com/26519/risks-essential-oilswellnessmama.com/26519/risks-essential-oils

Taking Charge at:

www.takingcharge.csh.umn.edu/explore-healing-practices/aromatherapy/are-essential-oils-safe

But of course, it is always advisable to speak to a health professional before using any of the products – especially if you have any concerns.

21 LITTLE KNOWN RECIPES FOR ALLERGY RELIEF

This chapter is going to give you some recipes for allergies that you can create in your own kitchen. Just remember all of the dilution and blending rules as you follow the instructions in the following pages.

1. Handmade Eczema Cream

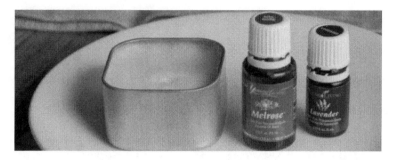

This recipe is great for sensitive skin. It's suitable for all ages, including babies.

Ingredients:

- 1/4 cup coconut oil (soft or melted)

- 1/4 cup shea butter

- 1/2 tsp. Vitamin E Oil

- 25 drops of Melrose Essential Oil

- 15 drops of Lavender Essential Oil

Directions:

In a small bowl, combine coconut oil, shea butter, and vitamin E oil. Stir or whisk well.

Add in essential oils, stir until well incorporated.

Transfer the cream to a container. You can store this at room temperature, but if your home is warm (above 76 degrees) it may get a little "melty." It will still do the trick but might be a little messy. If this is the case, simply store in the refrigerator.

Makes about 4 oz of cream. It's for topical application on the affected area.

2. Serum for Dark Circles

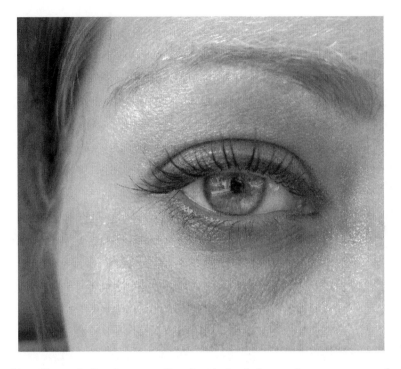

A side effect of allergies can often be dark circles under your eyes – from lack of sleep and feeling under the weather. Below is a great solution for this. This recipe is for adult usage.

Ingredients:

- 20 drops of Lavender Essential Oil

- 15 drops of Roman Chamomile Essential Oil

- 10 drops of Frankincense Essential Oil

- Rosehip Oil (organic)

- Sweet Almond Oil (organic)

Supplies:

- 5 ml glass bottle

- 1 roller fitment

- Stainless Steel Mini Funnel

Directions:

- In the clean 5 ml bottle, add the essential oils, then the carrier oils. You're aiming for 50% Almond Oil and 50% Rose Hips Oil. After you've secured the fitment top on the bottle, roll it between your hands gently to mix the solution.

- You can use this 2-3 times daily on your eyes by rolling it along the outside of your eye, and then lightly massaging it into your skin for about a minute.

- CAUTION: Be careful not to get this directly into your eyes! If you do, then flush your eyes with carrier oil – *not* water.

3. Sinus Headache Blends

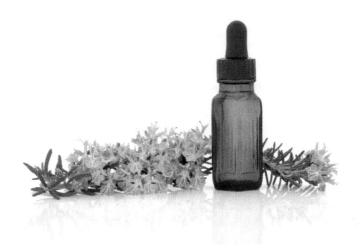

Here are two great blends for ridding yourself of the headaches that often come with allergies. These blends are for adult users and are for topical application.

Headache-Be-Gone Compress

Ingredients:

- 5 drops lavender or eucalyptus oil

- 1 cup cold water

Directions:

Add essential oil to water, and swish a soft cloth in it. Wring out the cloth, lie down, and close your eyes. Place the cloth over your forehead and eyes. Use throughout the day, as often as you can.

Migraine Headache Hand Soak

Ingredients:

- 5 drops lavender oil

- 5 drops ginger oil

- 1 quart hot water, about 110F

Directions:

Add essential oils to the hot water, and soak hands for at least 3 minutes. This therapy can be done repeatedly.

4. Relief for Peanut Anaphylactic Shock

Here is a great selection of essential oils for anaphylactic shock, which is recommended by a sufferer. It isn't exactly a recipe, more of a first aid kit that you should always have to hand:

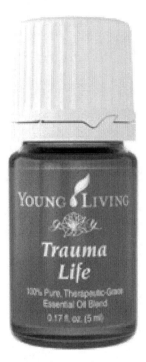

- Trauma Life for the shock.

- Valor to get you grounded.

- Purification to clear your system and stop the itching.

- RC for when you get congested.

- Frankincense for your immune system.

- Di-Gize can be applied for your stomach for nausea.

5. A Hay Fever Bath

Hay fever symptoms can be relieved by using the following guide. It's for aromatic use and is suitable for all ages.

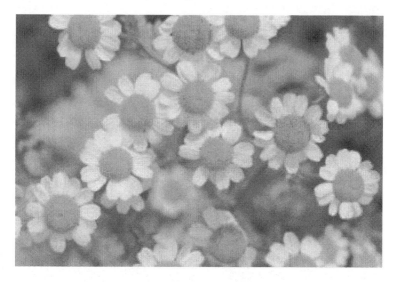

Ingredients:

- Roman Chamomile

- Lemon

- Eucalyptus globules

- Lavender

Directions:

When the seasonal allergy starts, try to infuse or inhale Roman Chamomile – just a drop per day. This usually lessens the reaction. Once you have a hay fever reaction, simply add a couple drops of Roman Chamomile, Lemon and Lavender to your bath, and relax. You can diffuse in the air too.

If you prefer to use a rub, just blend the above with a tablespoon of carrier oil and apply to your neck or chest. Refer to the <u>Dilution</u> chapter of this book for more information on how to get this blend to suit your needs.

6. 'Allergies Be Gone' Diffuser Mix

Here is an essential oil blend to use in your diffuser to help relieve the symptoms of allergies. These oils can be diluted to suit your needs. Refer to the <u>Dilution</u> chapter of this book to ensure the blend is right for you, and the age of people in your home.

- 2 drops Peppermint

- 2 drops Lemon

- 2 drops Lavender

Add this blend to 80ml of water and then put in the diffuser.

Alternatively you can place 1-2 drops of each of the 3 oils in a shot glass with water and gargle for a few minutes before swallowing. Or add all 3 oils in a tablespoon of raw honey and swallow for instant relief.

7. Sinus Congestion Blend

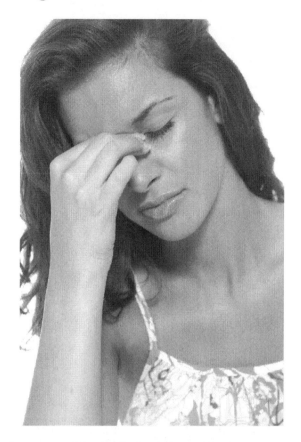

Below are three great blends for assisting with sinus congestion, which stops you from breathing, gives you headache and drive you insane. These are for adult usage and to be taken aromatically.

Ingredients:

- 2 drops Eucalyptus

- 2 drops Peppermint

- 2 drops Tea Tree

Directions:

- Boil a pot of water and remove it from the stove.

- While it is still steaming, add 2 drops peppermint, 2 drops eucalyptus and 2 drops of tea tree. Immediately cover the pot and head with a towel and inhale for 3 minutes.

- Keep eyes closed.

Blend #2

Ingredients:

- 25 drops Balsam fir

- 25 drops Eucalyptus dives

- 15 drops Laurel leaf

- 40 drops Tea Tree

Directions:

- In a glass orifice reducer bottle, blend the essential oils undiluted for an inhale or steam.

- To do steam, add one drop of this blend to a bowl of steamy water. Make sure the water is just steaming, not boiling.

- Close your eyes, lean over the bowl and breathe in the oil. To enhance the effect, use towel over your head to create a tent.

- Do this steam two times a day for a week. Then take a break for a few days and do it again twice a day for another week.

Blend #3

Ingredients:

- Eucalyptus essential oil

- Cypress essential oil

- Tea tree oil

Directions:

- Use 4-5 drops of eucalyptus oil, 4-5 drops of tea tree oil and 2-3 drops of cypress oil in a bowl of hot water.

- Cover your head with towel and breathe in.

- Keep your eyes closed.

8. Sleepy Spray

Allergies can affect every aspect of your life, and sleep is a huge factor in this. If you're having trouble, here are great recipes for this. These recipes are suitable for adults.

Ingredients:

- Almost 2 ounces of Ancient Minerals magnesium oil.

- 20 drops Peace&Calming or Lavender, Cedarwood, or Roman Chamomile essential oil. (Refer to the <u>Dilution</u> chapter of this book if you want to adjust this to suit you).

Supplies:

- 2-ounce dark glass spray bottle.

Directions:

- Fill your spray bottle with Ancient Minerals magnesium oil.

- Add your essential oils.

- Put on spray cap and shake bottle well.

- Apply to feet and rub in 20 minutes before bed. Also, cup hands and inhale oil residue for added benefit.

Blend #2

Ingredients:

- 3 drops of Lavender

- 1 drop Clary sage

Directions:

- Mix these essential oils in a teaspoon of milk or cream. Add to warm bath and soak.

9. Herpes Remedy

Here is a very effective essential oil blend for the herpes virus. This recipe is for adult usage and is for topical application.

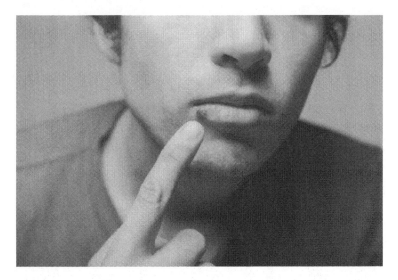

Ingredients:

- 10 drops tea tree oil

- 5 drops myrrh oil

- 5 drops geranium or bergamot oil

- 2 drops peppermint oil (optional)

- 1/2-ounce vegetable oil (any carrier oil)

Directions:

Combine the ingredients (refer to the <u>Dilution</u> chapter of this book if you wish to jig the recipe to suit your needs) and shake or stir well. Apply directly to affected area three to five times a day during an outbreak. The peppermint oil is optional because some people find it increases, rather than dulls, the pain. If you would prefer a less oily formula, you can substitute either rubbing alcohol or vodka for the vegetable oil, but try a little first to make sure the alcohol doesn't sting too much.

10. Hives Recipes

Hives are the red, itchy patches of skin that appear as a result of allergies. There are several different options for using essential oils to get rid of hives. These recipes are for adult usage (but can be adjusted to suit your needs via the Dilution chapter of this book) and is for topical application.

Hives Skin Wash

Ingredients:

- 5 drops chamomile or 10 drops lavender oil

- 2 drops peppermint oil

- 3 tablespoons baking soda

- 2 cups water (or use peppermint tea instead)

Directions:

Combine the ingredients. If you are making a tea to use as the base instead of water, pour 21/2 cups of boiling water over 4 teaspoons of dried peppermint leaves, and steep 15 minutes. Strain out the herb. Add the remaining ingredients. Use a soft cloth or a skin sponge to apply on irritated skin until itching is alleviated. Chamomile is the best choice for this recipe, but it is expensive, so 10 drops of lavender essential oil can be substituted, if necessary.

Hives Paste

Ingredients:

- 1/4 cup of the Hives Skin Wash (above)

- 3 tablespoons bentonite clay

Directions:

Stir the ingredients into a paste, and wait about five minutes for it to thicken. Apply to irritated skin with your fingers or a wooden tongue depressor. Let dry on skin, and leave for at least 45 minutes before washing off. Reapply for another 30 minutes if the area is still itching.

Hives wash blend

Ingredients:

- Lavender essential oil

- Chamomile essential oil

- Almond oil (optional)

Directions:

- Combine 10-15 drops of Chamomile essential oil and Lavender essential oil in 20oz of water. Soak a washcloth in the mixture and gently wipe the affected areas for immediate relief.

- Alternatively you can mix the essential oils with a carrier oil such as almond oil and apply this on the area where you have hives.

11. Post Natal Drip Syndrome Recipe

Post-nasal drip is the sensation of mucus accumulating or dripping in the back of your throat. Post-nasal drip can irritate your throat, causing a sore throat or cough. It can go along with a stuffy nose if you have a nasal allergy or a cold. Below is a great blend for this, which is for adult usage and to be applied topically.

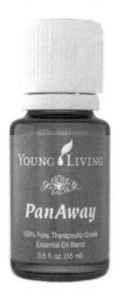

Ingredients:

- Panaway (You can make your own using the following ingredients if you wish wintergreen, helichrysum, clove and peppermint. If you do this, refer to the <u>Dilution</u> chapter of this guide to get the blend right)

- V6 Carrier Oil (or Olive Oil)

Directions:

- Mix 1-3 drops of the essential oil to 1 tsp of carrier oil.

- Apply through self-massage of area(s) where your discomfort lies, being careful to keep the oils away from your eyes. You can also massage the neurolymphatic points and foot reflex points that correlate to areas of the body that are troubling you.

12. Relief for Sensitive Irritated Eyes

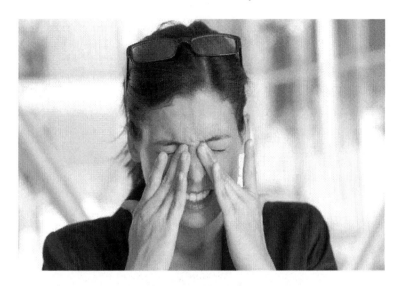

Here is a great recipe for helping with eye irritation, which is for adult usage but can be changed to suit your needs by using the <u>Dilution</u> chapter of this guide. It's to be applied topically.

Ingredients:

- Roman Chamomile Essential Oil

- Frankincense Essential Oil

- Lavender Essential Oil

- Almond Oil

Directions:

- Combine 5 drops of lavender, 4 drops of roman chamomile, 3 drops of frankincense and a teaspoon of almond oil.

- Put this into a small glass bottle with a roller top, then you can roll it around your eyes when you feel the itching for instant relief.

13. Oils to Diffuse for Mould Allergies

Diffusing certain essential oils can get rid of spores in your home. Here is a list of the best options. This is suitable for any age, but be very careful with children (The <u>Essential Oils to Avoid</u> chapter has more information about this). The oils can be used individually, or 2 or 3 can be combined to make a blend. If you wish to do this, refer to the <u>Dilution</u> chapter of this guide for more information on how to ensure the options suit you.

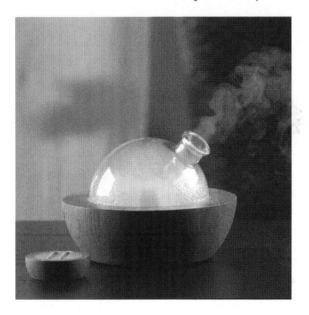

Options:

- Cinnamon

- Melaleuca (tea tree)

- Oregano

- Clove

- Thyme

- Grapefruit extract

- Rosemary

14. Pet Hair Allergies Essential Oils

Below is a list of essential oils that are great to use in a diffuser to help with pet hair allergies. These aromatic options are suitable for any age, but be very careful with children (The Essential Oils to Avoid chapter has more information about this). Refer to the Dilution chapter of this guide for more information on how to ensure the options suit you.

Options:

- Lavender

- Peppermint

- Roman Chamomile

- Lemon

- Eucalyptus

Or the combination of Lemon, Peppermint and Lavender. This blend is the best way to tackle most allergic reactions. Combined, they work as one of the most powerful antihistamines to bring down inflammation and other discomforts caused by your body's allergic response.

15. Lactose Intolerance Assistance

Dairy allergy is a common one, and here is a brilliant selection of blends for adult usage to help with it. If you want to change any of these recipes to suit your needs, refer to the <u>Dilution</u> chapter of this book.

Everyday Relief:

Ingredients:

- Lemon Oil

- Peppermint Oil

- Water

Directions:

Add 1-2 drops lemon oil or 1-2 drops Peppermint oil to 8-12oz of drinking water and drink it throughout the day.

Immediate Relief:

Ingredients:

- Lemon Oil

Directions:

For immediate relief of Lactose symptoms take 2-3 drops of Lemon essential oil, on the tongue and swish it in the mouth for 1 minute, then swallow. The Lemon will help neutralize the stomach acids and relieve pain.

Foot Rub

Ingredients:

- Peppermint Oil

- Marjoram Oil

- Dill

Directions:

Rub 3-4 drops of Peppermint, Marjoram or Dill essential oils, or all three oils, onto the abdomen or soles of feet.

Herbal Tea

Ingredients:

- Peppermint Oil

- Marjoram Oil

- Dill

- Water

- Honey

Directions:

Mix 1 drop of Peppermint oil and 1 drop Marjoram or Dill essential oil into a teaspoon of honey, add it to half or full cup of warm water.

For Cramping

Ingredients:

- Fennel oil

- Honey

- Water

- V6 Carrier Oil

Directions

Fennel is primarily beneficial for the digestive system. It helps relieve abdominal cramping. Take 2-3 drops in a capsule, then fill with carrier oil, or add 2-3 drops to 1 tsp. honey, added to half or full cup of warm water for a nice herbal tea. Fennel relieves flatulence, assists with constipation and stagnation, and Neutralizes toxicity of the body.

Digestion Blend

Ingredients:

- Coriander

- Dill

- Peppermint

- Fennel

- Ginger Root

- Lemon

- V6 Carrier Oil

Directions:

Rub 3-4 drops of each essential oils mixed with a carrier oil over the abdomen or soles of feet. Can also ingest 1-2 drops, as needed.

16. A Blend to Help You Breathe

A congested or runny nose is one of the most common symptoms of allergies. These blends are also great for adult asthma sufferers. It will help you relax and open airways and tissues of the nose, throat, and lungs. It's for aromatic usage and can be changed to suit your personal needs using the Dilution chapter of this guide.

Ingredients:

- 30 drops Ravensara

- 45 drops Eucalyptus Globulus (use Eucalyptus Radiata for children)

- 18 drops Lemon

- 16 drops Tea Tree (Melaleuca)

- 10 drops Laurel Leaf

- 5 drops Peppermint

Directions:

Put this mix into an empty clean EO dropper bottle. Cap and shake for 2 minutes. Label and its ready to use!

Blend #2

Ingredients:

- 2 drops Eucalyptus Globulus (use Eucalyptus Radiata for children)

- 2 drops Lemon

- 2 drops Tea Tree (Melaleuca)

- 2 drops Peppermint

- Almond oil (optional)

Directions:

Mix two drops of each of peppermint, eucalyptus, tea tree and lemon essential oils. Use this steam for inhalation or in a diffuser.

To apply this blend to your skin, use the same amounts of essential oils as for inhalation, but mix this blend with an ounce of almond oil. Rub this into your chest and around collarbones and inhale.

17. Rash

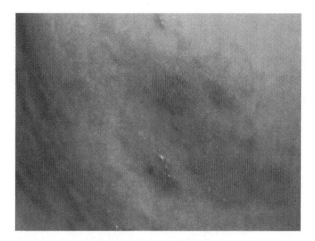

Here are a few essential oil treatments for rashes. They can be used for any age, but be careful with very young children. Refer to the Dilution chapter of the book for more information.

Bath

Ingredients:

- Lavender

- Chamomile

- Eucalyptus

Directions:

Add a few drops of lavender oil, chamomile oil and eucalyptus oil to your bath water. Soak in this tub bath for 20 minutes. (If you have only one of these oils, simply use that standalone.)

Serum

Ingredients:

- Baking Soda

- Lavender

Directions:

Alternatively, mix baking soda with few drops of lavender essential oil. Apply the mixture all over the rash until it is completely covered. This essential oil remedy for heat rash can even be used on babies and infants. When treating baby for prickly heat using these essential oil remedies, make sure that its skin is kept completely dry, especially in the folds of skin.

For babies under the age of 2 years, use only quarter cup of baking soda to which 2-3 drops of lavender oil are added. For older kids (up to 7 years), you can use more soda and oil respectively. For adults, use about a cup of soda and 5-8 drops of lavender oil.

Alternatively, if you are able to get fresh neem leaves, simply boil a handful of those leaves and add the extracts to the bath water. Neem has antibacterial properties and can prevent secondary skin infections arising from prickly heat rashes.

TIP: **How to relief from itching when there is no rash?**

Often allergies cause itching even when there is no visible rash.

Simply dilute 2-3 drops of Lavender and Peppermint essential oil in an ounce of Almond oil, and gently spread this across the areas that begin to itch.

18. Essential Oil Inhaler

Here is a brilliant way of creating your very own inhaler, using essential oils. This is for aromatic usage and is suitable for adults.

Ingredients:

- 4 drops Balsam Fir essential oil

- 3 drops Peppermint essential oil

- 3 drops Eucalyptus globulus essential oil

- 5 drops Frankincense Essential Oil

Directions:

Add these oils to the cotton part of a blank inhaler.

19. Immune Tonic Blend

Allergies can have a massive impact on your immune system, and this blend is great for boosting you internally. This is for adult usage and can be edited if needed by using the <u>Dilution</u> chapter of this guide.

Ingredients:

- 6 drops lavender oil

- 6 drops bergamot oil

- 3 drops lemon oil

- 3 drops tea tree oil

- 2 drops myrrh oil (optional)

- 2 ounces' vegetable oil

Directions:

Combine ingredients. Use as a general massage oil or over specific areas of the body that tend to develop physical problems. For example, if you come down with a lot of chest colds and flus, rub this blend over your chest. Use 1 to 2 teaspoons in a bath or 1 teaspoon in a foot bath. Without the vegetable oil, this recipe is suitable for use in an aromatherapy diffuser, simmering pan of water, or potpourri cooker. Use in some form several times a day when trying to build up your own natural immunity.

20. Blend for Intestinal Ailments

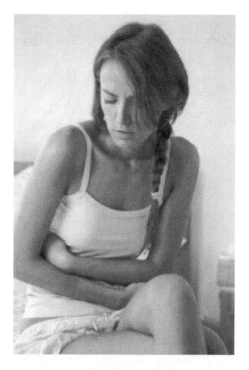

Below is a great recipe for internal discomfort, which can be caused by food allergies. The blend below is for adult usage, but can be changed by using the <u>Dilution</u> chapter of this guide, and is to be used topically.

Ingredients:

- 1 drop Peppermint oil

- 1 drop Chamomile oil

- 2 drops Rosemary oil

- 1 drop Clove oil

Directions:

Blend with 5 ml vegetable carrier oil and rub on your belly, over the area of discomfort.

21. Atopic Dermatitis Blend

Here is a brilliant blend for helping with atopic dermatitis. It's for adult usage, but can be changed to suit specific needs by using the <u>Dilution</u> chapter of this book.

Ingredients:

- 4 drops Frankincense

- 3 drops Cedarwood

- 3 drops German Chamomile

- 4 drops Lavender

- 3 drops Helichrysum

- 3 drops Rosemary

- 10ml of Coconut oil

- 10ml of Meadowfoam seed oil

- 5ml Jojoba oil

- 4ml Rosehip oil

Directions:

Add the essential oil drops to the carrier oil in a 30 ml container. Calendula Supercritical extract can be added at 0.5% or 2 drops per ounce. Then this blend is ready to be applied topically to the affected area.

2 MOST COMMON MISTAKES FOR ESSENTIAL OIL USE

Below are the two most common mistakes in the use of essential oils, and suggestions on how to avoid them:

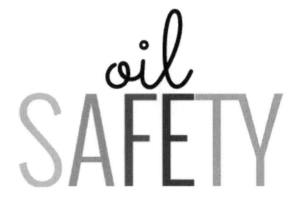

1. Essential oil overdose: Using too much, too often.

If you're a regular user of essential oils, there is a good chance that you are also someone who prefers to put very little medication in your body. You understand that when you put a medication in your body, the medication needs to be detoxified through your liver or kidney systems. This detox process takes time and can be hard work for your liver and kidneys, many times causing toxicity side effects.

The same is true for essential oils. In no way do essential oils have the same side effects, but just like a medication, each person's constitution is different and will respond differently to essential oils and the amount you use. To avoid overusing essential oils, it is recommended to approach essential oils thoughtfully and sparingly.

2. Unbalanced use of essential oils

Some essential oils are heating to the body and some are cooling. For example, during the winter, a person should use less peppermint essential oils (or other mint oils). Because mint oils are very cooling, they can do an excellent job to calm down the digestive system, but if overused during the winter, it can really mess up your digestion long term.

On the other hand, if a person uses something like clove or cinnamon oil, these are both warming. If you are someone who already has a warm constitution or has too much internal heat, using too many warming essential oils could cause hormonal, headache, blood pressure or heart problems. Women, or even men, can develop hot flashes from using too many warming oils. These warming essential oils need time to properly clear through the liver. Unwanted symptoms from warming oils can especially pop up during the summer months.

The goal with essential oils is to use them in a balanced way by appropriately using cooling and warming oils together.

It's also advisable to refer to the <u>Safety</u> chapter of this book before using essential oils, and to speak to a health professional if you have any questions.

RESOURCES

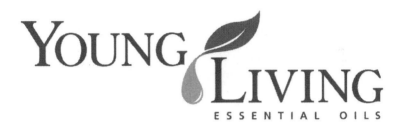

www.youngliving.com

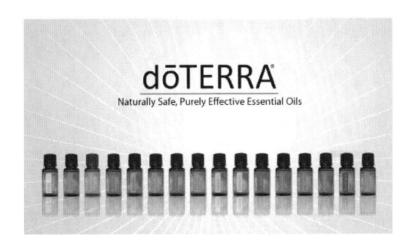

www.doterra.com

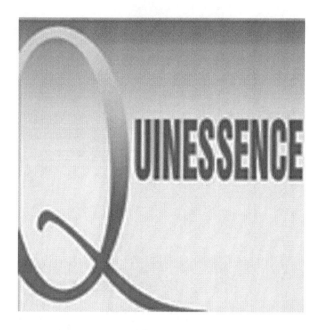

www.quinessence.com

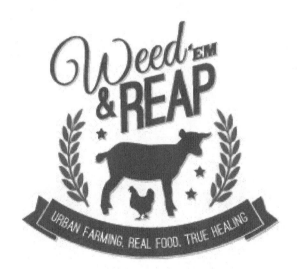

www.weedemandreap.com

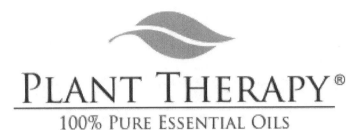

www.planttherapy.com

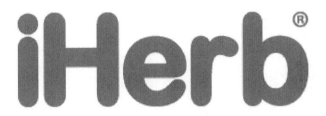

www.iherb.com

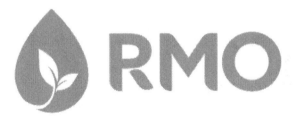

www.rockymountainoils.com

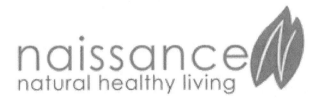

www.enaissance.co.uk

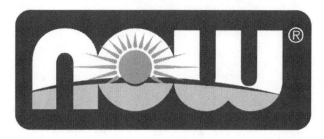

Nutrition for Optimal Wellness™

www.nowfoods.com

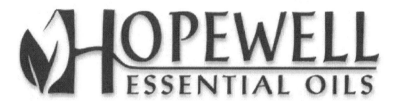

hopewelloils.com

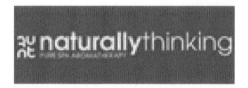

www.naturallythinking.com

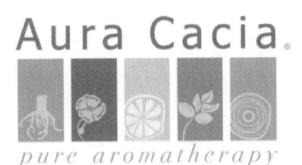

www.auracacia.com

 Native American Nutritionals

www.nativeamericannutritionals.com

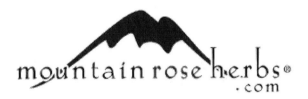

www.mountainroseherbs.com

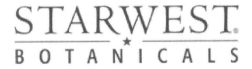

www.starwest-botanicals.com

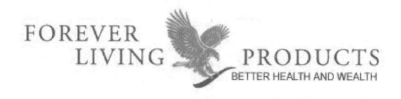

foreverliving.com

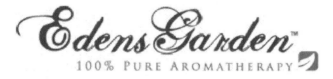

www.edensgarden.com

FAQ

1. Which essential oils are safe to use if you are pregnant?

The <u>Pregnancy</u> section in this book goes into more detail on this subject. Essential oils can affect hormones, gut bacteria and other aspects of health and extreme care should be used when taking them while pregnant or nursing. It is suggested that the essential oils that appear to be safe to use during pregnancy include:

- Cardamon

- Frankincense

- Geranium

- Neroli

- Patchouli

- Petitgrain

- Rosewood

- Rose

- Sandalwood

- And other nontoxic essential oils.

2. Is price an indicator of an essential oil's quality?

As stated in the <u>Pure vs. Quality</u> chapter in this book:

"Pure means undiluted, whereas quality refers to how well the product is made. There can be a bad quality oil, that's pure."

The reputation and standards of the company that has made the oil, is a *much* better indicator of the product you will be buying.

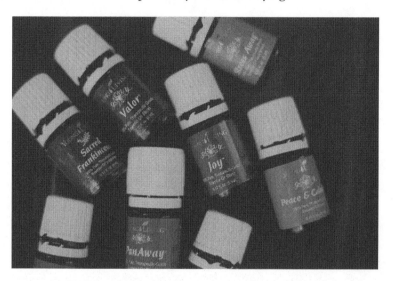

3. How do I know if an essential oil companies marketing is deceptive?

Some companies, however unintentionally, will use terms such as *'therapeutic grade'*, *'medicinal grade'* or *'aromatherapy grade'*. These companies may not be trying to mislead you, but that is what they are doing all the same.

If you *do* come across these titles on the labels of essential oils, you need to examine the key ingredients to judge for yourself the quality. This might be difficult when you are just starting out using these oils, so you can always research the company's reputation. The Internet is a great resource for this, you can even ask the opinions of other users, on forums such as <u>myessentialoilsforum.com</u>.

4. Which essential oils can be toxic in certain conditions?

You need to be careful with using essential oils if you're very old, very young or pregnant. <u>Aromatherapy Bible</u> (<u>aromatherapybible.com/toxicity-of-essential-oils</u>) has a great, in-depth guide on this subject if you require more information.

5. How can essential oils soothe itchy, watery eyes caused by allergies?

The following essential oils are suggested for itchy, watery eyes:

- Lavender

- Peppermint

- Lemon

- Eucalyptus

- Roman Chamomile

In general, lavender essential oil is the most effective oil for helping your eyes.

6. How can essential oils help to open up your airways?

The <u>recipe</u> chapter of this book gives a few good examples of essential oil blends that can help with this. There is also *Breathe Again* from Young Living to consider as an option.

Breathe Again
Benefits and Everyday Uses

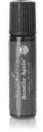

I use with R.C and Raven for added benefits!

Coughs
Bronchitis
Stuffy Noses
Sinusitis
Immune Support
Supports Lung Health

Promotes healthy Sinus Function
Reduces Localized Discomfort

Contains:
4 Eucalyptus Oils
Laurus Nobilis
Peppermint
Copaiba
Myrtle
Rose Hip
Blue Cypress
Coconut Oil

*Apply to feet to boost immune system
*Apply generously to chest and throat
*Diffuse or breath in aroma

7. How can essential oils eliminate some common allergens?

The main essential oil blend that is considered to assist with all allergies is Lavender, Lemon and Peppermint. These oils help to maintain feelings of clear airways and easy breathing. These three oils together can help minimize the effects of seasonal threats. Lavender works as a natural antihistamine and process strong anti-inflammatory properties to treat and relief most allergic reactions. Peppermint is very effective to treat respiratory or digestive issues because it has pain-relieving, soothing, cooling and anti-inflammatory properties. Lemon works as a natural antihistamine, relieves excess mucus, and cools down the inflammation.

Simply add 1-3 drops of each to shot glass of juice or water, swish 10-20 seconds in the mouth and swallow.

8. Why is it so difficult to find pure therapeutic grade essential oil?

It is because it takes hundreds of pounds of materials to make a pound of pure therapeutic grade oil. For example, it takes 30 – 60 roses to make one single drop of it! Unfortunately, companies often take short cuts to save money, so you will need to do your research to ensure you're getting what you want. Note that a bottle only has to have 10% of the actual oil in it to be considered 100% pure!

9. What is the difference between Aromatherapy and Essential Oil Therapy?

Aromatherapy is the practice of using essential oils, so Essential Oil Therapy is simply another way of saying the same thing.

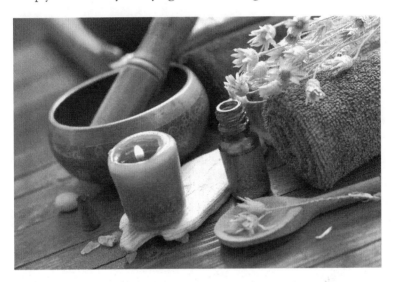

10. Which essential oils should be avoided and why?

The 'Essential Oils To Avoid' chapter looks into this in detail. However, finding out the oils *you* should avoid can be discovered by trial and error and talking to a health professional. Everyone is unique and has individual needs.

11. Where are most common places for buying essential oil blends?

You will be able to buy essential oils from your local health care store, and there are also many online Resources at your fingertips.

12. Are there any clinical studies to prove the healing properties of essential oils?

As essential oils rise in popularity, the number of studies being done increases. Most of the data from this can be found at the *NCBI* website (www.ncbi.nlm.nih.gov/pubmedhealth/PMH0032645).

13. If I have perfume allergies can I use essential oils?

It is advisable to look for neutral or scent free products if you suffer from a perfume allergies. *Naturally Thinking* (www.naturallythinking.com) has a large range of these.

14. Are essential oils bad for people who have tree allergies?

If you suffer from tree allergies, you *can* struggle with essential oils. It is always advised to do a Patch Test on your skin to check that you'll be ok.

15. What essential oil can I use to safely drain my sinuses from serious allergies?

Oregano oil is suggested as a remedy for draining sinuses:

- Mix 1 drop Oregano oil and 2 ounces of carrier oil, apply externally along sinus areas of the face (avoid the eyes)

- Apply Oil mixture on tips of fingers. Beginning at top of nose, above the eyes, run fingers along sinus passages, behind jaw and down throat.

- Next, apply Oil mixture to tips of fingers, beginning at bridge of nose, run fingers under eyes, on upper cheek, behind jaw line and down throat. Apply a gentle pressure each time.

- If you are congested at all, you will notice that you need to swallow or sniff, as mucus is being moved around and thinned in your sinus passage and is triggering a response to get rid of it. Don't sniff and pull it back into the sinuses.

- Perform the same motion a few more times, then blow your nose.

- Take great care not to get oil mixture in eye.

- Use the oil by inhaling the same mixture as often as needed to open up clogged sinuses.

- In extreme cases, take a capsule with 2 drops Oregano, filled with carrier oil, internally 2 times daily.

You may also look at the <u>Sinus congestion</u> recipes described in this guide.

16. Are there any essential oils that relieve itching?

Here's a great recipes to relieve itching:

Fill a 2-ounce spray bottle to the shoulder with witch hazel.

Add the following essential oils:

- 5 drops Lavender

- 2 drops Frankincense

- 3 drops Tea Tree

Label your bottle, shake it up, and use – that's it!

CONCLUSION

So as you can see from all of the information in this book, using essential oils to help fight and prevent your allergies is a safer, more natural and with many less side effects that traditional medicine.

The benefits of essential oils are:

- **Non toxic** – these oils are all natural, there is nothing toxic that can harm you if you use them correctly.

- **Easy to use** – they can be used wherever you are, and the methods necessary to take the oils are very simple.

- **Very Powerful** – Essential Oils can have a healing effect mentally, physically, and emotionally.

So there really is no reason to not *at least* give them a try!

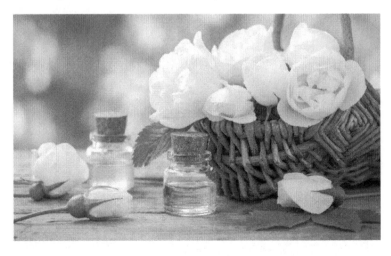

Now that you have all the information that you need to get yourself started with using essential oils, there is nothing holding you back. With all the online resources, you can also continue doing your own research into possible products that you may go on to use.

It's highly recommended to use online forums to speak to other essential oil users, as you can get a wealth of information from them. Here are some forums to get you started:

The Aromatherapy Place at auroma.forumchitchat.com

Ananda Apocthecary at www.anandaapothecary.com/forums

Essential Oil Goddess at www.essential-oil-goddess.com/aromatherapy-forum.html

Of course, it is always recommended to speak to a health professional before using any oils to check that they will suit you.

ABOUT THE AUTHOR

Mary Jones became interested in herbal remedies early on in her life. She came to essential oils after years of looking for solutions to her problems in the medical world. Issues like allergies, weight loss, and lack of energy didn't really seem to have good solutions in the traditional medicine. There were expensive treatments to be had, but often they did not work in the long term and were not as holistic as Mary wanted the treatments to be.

In her search for a solution, she came upon essential oils and aromatherapy. As she had learned about the stress relieving power of aromatherapy, she began intensely studying essential oils–how they work, how they are used, how they are made, which are safe to use, and beyond. She travelled to study with those who had long used essential oils and taught others about the many uses. For decades, she has developed her knowledge about this subject.

One of Mary's life goals is to make the world a better, happier place, and her writings are definitely a testament to that. She has not just kept all of her research and discoveries to herself. She has elected to share them, in a format that makes them available to just about everyone.

Now, after years of compiling information about the most beneficial and useful essential oils, Mary has written several books to introduce others to the knowledge she has gathered.

Made in the USA
Las Vegas, NV
04 November 2023

80253419R00134